SUMMARY REPORT 2007

National Asthma Education and Prevention Program
Expert Panel Report 3

Guidelines for the Diagnosis and Management of Asthma

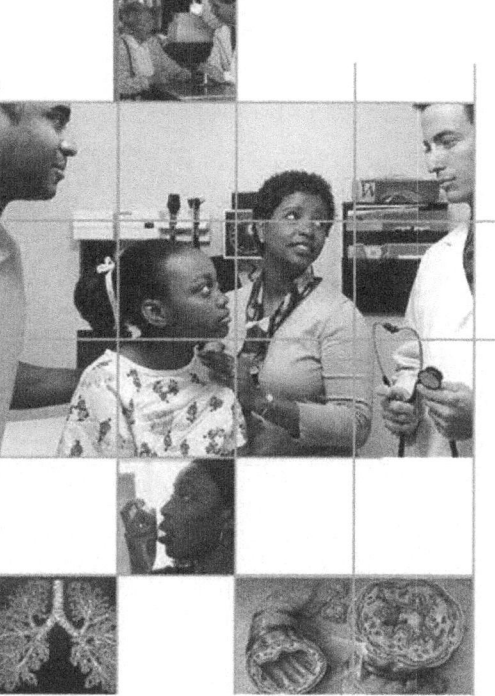

U.S. Department of Health and Human Services
National Institutes of Health

National **Heart**
Lung and Blood Institute

NIH Publication Number 08-5846
October 2007

Contents

Acknowledgments	iii
Preface	ix
Introduction	1
Asthma Definition and Implications for Treatment	9
Definition and Pathophysiology	9
Causes of Asthma	10
Implications for Treatment	10
Diagnosis of Asthma	11
Managing Asthma Long Term	15
Four Components of Asthma Care	15
Component 1: Assessing and Monitoring Asthma Severity and Asthma Control	15
Component 2: Education for a Partnership in Care	18
Component 3: Control of Environmental Factors and Comorbid Conditions That Affect Asthma	23
Allergens and Irritants	23
Comorbid Conditions	25
Component 4: Medications	28
General Mechanisms and Role in Therapy	28
Delivery Devices for Inhaled Medications	29
Safety Issues for Inhaled Corticosteroids and Long-Acting Beta$_2$-Agonists	29
Inhaled Corticosteroids	29
Inhaled Corticosteroids and Linear Growth in Children	30
Long-Acting Beta$_2$-Agonists	30
Stepwise Approach for Managing Asthma	30
Principles of the Stepwise Approach	30
Stepwise Treatment Recommendations for Different Ages	34
Steps for Children 0–4 Years of Age	34
Steps for Children 5–11 Years of Age	35
Steps for Youths >12 Years of Age and Adults	37
Managing Special Situations	38
Exercise-Induced Bronchospasm	38
Pregnancy	38
Surgery	39
Disparities	39
Managing Exacerbations	53
Classifying Severity	53
Home Management	53
Management in the Urgent or Emergency Care and Hospital Settings	54
For More Information	back cover

List of Boxes and Figures

Figure 1.	Summary of Recommended Key Clinical Activities for the Diagnosis and Management of Asthma	4
Figure 2.	The Interplay and Interaction Between Airway Inflammation and the Clinical Symptoms and Pathophysiology of Asthma	9
Figure 3.	Suggested Items for Medical History*	13
Figure 4.	Sample Patient Self-Assessment Sheet for Followup Visits*	17
Figure 5.	Asthma Action Plan—Adult	20
Figure 6.	Sample Asthma Action Plan—Child	21
Figure 7.	Delivery of Asthma Education by Clinicians During Patient Care Visits	22
Figure 8.	Asthma Education Resources	24
Figure 9.	How To Control Things That Make Your Asthma Worse	26
Figure 10.	Aerosol Delivery Devices	31
Figure 11.	Classifying Asthma Severity and Initiating Therapy in Children	40
Figure 12.	Assessing Asthma Control and Adjusting Therapy in Children	41
Figure 13.	Stepwise Approach for Managing Asthma Long Term in Children, 0–4 Years of Age and 5–11 Years of Age	42
Figure 14.	Classifying Asthma Severity and Initiating Treatment in Youths ≥12 Years of Age and Adults	43
Figure 15.	Assessing Asthma Control and Adjusting Therapy in Youths ≥12 Years of Age and Adults	44
Figure 16.	Stepwise Approach for Managing Asthma in Youths ≥12 Years of Age and Adults	45
Figure 17.	Usual Dosages for Long-term control Medications*	46
Figure 18.	Estimated Comparative Daily Dosages for Inhaled Corticosteroids	49
Figure 19.	Usual Dosages for Quick-Relief Medications*	50
Figure 20.	Classifying Severity of Asthma Exacerbations in the Urgent or Emergency Care Setting	54
Figure 21.	Management of Asthma Exacerbations: Emergency Department and Hospital-Based Care	55
Figure 22.	Dosages of Drugs for Asthma Exacerbations	56
Figure 23a.	Emergency Department—Asthma Discharge Plan	59
Figure 23b.	Emergency Department—Asthma Discharge Plan: How to Use Your Metered-Dose Inhaler	60

Acknowledgements

National Asthma Education and Prevention Program Coordinating Committee

Agency for Healthcare Research and Quality
Denise Dougherty, Ph.D.

Allergy & Asthma Network Mothers of Asthmatics
Nancy Sander

American Academy of Allergy, Asthma, and Immunology
Michael Schatz, M.D., M.S.

American Academy of Family Physicians
Kurtis S. Elward, M.D., M.P.H., F.A.A.F.P.

American Academy of Pediatrics
Gary S. Rachelefsky, M.D.

American Academy of Physician Assistants
Tera Crisalida, P.A.-C., M.P.A.S.

American Association for Respiratory Care
Thomas J. Kallstrom, R.R.T., F.A.A.R.C., AE-C

American College of Allergy, Asthma, and Immunology
William Storms, M.D.

American College of Chest Physicians
John Mitchell, M.D., F.A.C.P.

American College of Emergency Physicians
Richard M. Nowak, M.D., M.B.A., F.A.C.E.P.

American Lung Association
Noreen M. Clark, Ph.D.

American Medical Association
Paul V. Williams, M.D.

American Nurses Association
Karen Huss, D.N.Sc., R.N., A.P.R.N.B.C., F.A.A.N., F.A.A.A.I.

American Pharmacists Association
Dennis M. Williams, Pharm.D.

American Public Health Association
Pamela J. Luna, Dr.P.H., M.Ed.

American School Health Association
Lani S. M. Wheeler, M.D., F.A.A.P., F.A.S.H.A.

American Society of Health-System Pharmacists
Kathryn V. Blake, Pharm.D.

American Thoracic Society
Stephen C. Lazarus, M.D.

Asthma and Allergy Foundation of America
Mo Mayrides

Council of State and Territorial Epidemiologists
Sarah Lyon-Callo, M.A., M.S.

National Association of School Nurses
Donna Mazyck, R.N., M.S., N.C.S.N.

National Black Nurses Association, Inc.
Susan B. Clark, R.N., M.N.

National Center for Chronic Disease Prevention, Centers for Disease Control and Prevention (CDC)
Sarah Merkle, M.P.H.

National Center for Environmental Health, CDC
Paul M. Garbe, M.D.

National Center for Health Statistics, CDC
Lara Akinbami, M.D.

National Institute for Occupational Safety and Health, CDC
Margaret Filios, S.M., R.N.

National Heart, Lung, and Blood Institute
National Institutes of Health (NIH)
Elizabeth Nabel, M.D.

National Heart, Lung, and Blood Institute
NIH, Ad Hoc Committee on Minority Populations
Ruth I. Quartey, Ph.D.

National Institute of Allergy and Infectious Diseases (NIAID), NIH
Peter J. Gergen, M.D., M.P.H.

National Institute of Environmental Health Sciences, NIH
Charles A. Wells, Ph.D.

National Medical Association
Michael Lenoir, M.D.

National Respiratory Training Center
Pamela Steele, M.S.N., C.P.N.P., AE-C

Society for Academic Emergency Medicine
Rita Cydulka, M.D., M.S.

Society for Public Health Education
Judith C. Taylor-Fishwick, M.Sc., AE-C

U.S. Department of Education
Dana Carr

U.S. Environmental Protection Agency
Indoor Environments Division
David Rowson, M.S.

U.S. Environmental Protection Agency
Office of Research and Development
Hillel S. Koren, Ph.D.

U.S. Food and Drug Administration
Robert J. Meyer, M.D.

Third Expert Panel on the Management of Asthma

William W. Busse, M.D., Chair
University of Wisconsin Medical School
Madison, Wisconsin

Homer A. Boushey, M.D.
University of California–San Francisco
San Francisco, California

Carlos A. Camargo, Jr., M.D., Dr.P.H.
Massachusetts General Hospital
Boston, Massachusetts

David Evans, Ph.D., A.E.-C,
Columbia University
New York, New York

Michael B. Foggs, M.D.
Advocate Health Centers
Chicago, Illinois

Susan L. Janson, D.N.Sc., R.N., A.N.P., F.A.A.N.
University of California–San Francisco
San Francisco, California

H. William Kelly, Pharm.D.
University of New Mexico Health Sciences Center
Albuquerque, New Mexico

Robert F. Lemanske, M.D.
University of Wisconsin Hospital and Clinics
Madison, Wisconsin

Fernando D. Martinez, M.D.
University of Arizona Medical Center
Tucson, Arizona

Robert J. Meyer, M.D.
U.S. Food and Drug Administration
Silver Spring, Maryland

Harold S. Nelson, M.D.
National Jewish Medical and Research Center
Denver, Colorado

Thomas A. E. Platts-Mills, M.D., Ph.D.
University of Virginia School of Medicine
Charlottesville, Virginia

Michael Schatz, M.D., M.S.
Kaiser-Permanente–San Diego
San Diego, California

Gail Shapiro, M.D.*
University of Washington
Seattle, Washington

Stuart Stoloff, M.D.
University of Nevada School of Medicine
Carson City, Nevada

Stanley J. Szefler, M.D.
National Jewish Medical and Research Center
Denver, Colorado

Scott T. Weiss, M.D., M.S.
Brigham and Women's Hospital
Boston, Massachusetts

Barbara P. Yawn, M.D., M.Sc.
Olmstead Medical Center
Rochester, Minnesota

Development of the guidelines was funded by the NHLBI, NIH. Expert Panel members completed financial disclosure forms, and the Expert Panel members disclosed relevant financial interests to each other prior to their discussions. Expert Panel members participated as volunteers and were compensated only for travel expenses related to the Expert Panel meetings. Financial disclosure information covering the 3-year period during which the guidelines were developed is provided for each Expert Panel member below.

Dr. Busse has served on the Speakers' Bureaus of GlaxoSmithKline, Merck, Novartis, and Pfizer; and on the Advisory Boards of Altana, Centocor, Dynavax, Genentech/Novartis, GlaxoSmithKline, Isis, Merck, Pfizer, Schering, and Wyeth. He has received funding/grant support for research projects from Astellas, Centocor, Dynavax, GlaxoSmithKline, Novartis, and Wyeth. Dr. Busse also has research support from the NIH.

Dr. Boushey has served as a consultant for Altana, Protein Design Lab, and Sumitomo. He has received honoraria from Boehringer-Ingelheim, Genentech, Merck, Novartis, and Sanofi Aventis, and funding/grant support for research projects from the NIH.

Dr. Camargo has served on the Speakers' Bureaus of AstraZeneca, GlaxoSmithKline, Merck, and Schering Plough; and as a consultant for AstraZeneca, Critical Therapeutics, Dey Laboratories, GlaxoSmithKline, MedImmune, Merck, Novartis, Praxair, Respironics, Schering Plough, Sepracor, and TEVA. He has received funding/grant support for research projects from a variety of Government agencies and not-for-profit foundations, as well as AstraZeneca, Dey Laboratories, GlaxoSmithKline, MedImmune, Merck, Novartis, and Respiromics.

Dr. Evans has received funding/grant support for research projects from the NHLBI.

Dr. Foggs has served on the Speakers' Bureaus of GlaxoSmithKline, Merck, Pfizer, Sepracor, and UCB Pharma; on the Advisory Boards of Alcon, Altana, AstraZeneca, Critical Therapeutics, Genentech,

GlaxoSmithKline, and IVAX, and as consultant for Merck and Sepracor. He has received funding/grant support for research projects from GlaxoSmithKline.

Dr. Janson has served on the Advisory Board of Altana, and as a consultant for Merck. She has received funding/grant support for research projects from the NHLBI.

Dr. Kelly has served on the Speakers' Bureaus of AstraZeneca and GlaxoSmithKline; and on the MAP Pharmaceuticals Advisory Boards of AstraZeneca, Merck, Novartis, and Sepracor.

Dr. Lemanske has served on the Speakers' Bureaus of GlaxoSmithKline and Merck, and as a consultant for AstraZeneca, Aventis, GlaxoSmithKline, Merck, and Novartis. He has received honoraria from Altana, and funding/grant support for research projects from the NHLBI and NIAID.

Dr. Martinez has served on the Advisory Board of Merck and as a consultant for Genentech, GlaxoSmithKline, and Pfizer. He has received honoraria from Merck.

Dr. Meyer has no relevant financial interests.

Dr. Nelson has served on the Speakers' Bureaus of AstraZeneca, GlaxoSmithKline, Pfizer, and Schering Plough; and as a consultant for Air Pharma, Altana Pharma US, Astellas, AstraZeneca, Curalogic, Dey Laboratories, Dynavax Technologies, Genentech/Novartis, GlaxoSmithKline, Inflazyme Pharmaceuticals, MediciNova, Protein Design Laboratories, Sanofi-Aventis, Schering Plough, and Wyeth Pharmaceuticals. He has received funding/grant support for research projects from Altana, Astellas, AstraZeneca, Behringer, Critical Therapeutics, Dey Laboratories, Epigenesis, Genentech, GlaxoSmithKline, IVAX, Medicinova, Novartis, Sanofi-Aventis, Schering Plough, Sepracor, TEVA, and Wyeth.

Dr. Platts-Mills has served on the Advisory Committee of Indoor Biotechnologies. He has received funding/grant support for a research project from Pharmacia Diagnostics.

Dr. Schatz has served on the Speakers' Bureaus of AstraZeneca, Genentech, GlaxoSmithKline, and Merck; and as a consultant for GlaxoSmithKline on an unbranded asthma initiative. He has received funding/grant support for research projects from GlaxoSmithKline, Merck, and Sanofi-Aventis.

---

* The NAEPP would like to acknowledge the contributions of Dr. Gail Shapiro, who served on the NAEPP Expert Panels from 1991 until her death in August 2006. She had a passion for improving asthma care and an unwavering commitment to develop evidence-based recommendations that would offer practical guidance for clinicians and patients to work together to achieve asthma control.

Dr. Shapiro* served on the Speakers' Bureaus of AstraZeneca, Genentech, GlaxoSmithKline, IVAX Laboratories, Key Pharmaceuticals, Merck, Pfizer Pharmaceuticals, Schering Corporation, UCB Pharma, and 3M; and as a consultant for Altana, AstraZeneca, Dey Laboratories, Genentech/Novartis, GlaxoSmithKline, ICOS, IVAX Laboratories, Merck, Sanofi-Aventis, and Sepracor. She received funding/grant support for research projects from Abbott, AstraZeneca, Boehringer Ingelheim, Bristol-Myers-Squibb, Dey Laboratories, Fujisawa Pharmaceuticals, Genentech, GlaxoSmithKline, Immunex, Key, Lederle, Lilly Research, MedPointe Pharmaceuticals, Medtronic Emergency Response Systems, Merck, Novartis, Pfizer, Pharmaxis, Purdue Frederick, Sanofi-Aventis, Schering, Sepracor, 3M Pharmaceuticals, UCB Pharma, and Upjohn Laboratories.

Dr. Stoloff has served on the Speakers' Bureaus of Alcon, Altana, AstraZeneca, Genentech, GlaxoSmithKline, Novartis, Pfizer, Sanofi Aventis, and Schering; and as a consultant for Alcon, Altana, AstraZeneca, Dey, Genentech, GlaxoSmithKline, Merck, Novartis, Pfizer, Sanofi Aventis, and Schering.

Dr. Szefler has served on the Advisory Boards of Altana, AstraZeneca, Genentech, GlaxoSmithKline, Merck, Novartis, and Sanofi Aventis; and as a consultant for Altana, AstraZeneca, Genentech, GlaxoSmithKline, Merck, Novartis, and Sanofi Aventis. He has received funding/grant support for a research project from Ross.

Dr. Weiss has served on the Advisory Board of Genentech, and as a consultant for Genentech and GlaxoSmithKline. He has received funding/grant support for research projects from GlaxoSmithKline.

Dr. Yawn has served on the Advisory Boards of Altana, AstraZeneca, Merck, Sanofi Aventis, and Schering Plough. She has received honoraria from Pfizer and Schering Plough, and funding/grant support for research projects from the Agency for Healthcare Research and Quality, the CDC, the NHLBI, Merck, and Schering Plough.

Consultant Reviewers

Financial disclosure information covering a 12 month period prior to the review of the guidelines is provided below for each consultant.

Andrea J. Apter, M.D., M.Sc.
University of Pennsylvania Medical Center
Philadelphia, Pennsylvania

Noreen M. Clark, Ph.D.
University of Michigan School of Public Health
Ann Arbor, Michigan

Anne Fuhlbrigge, M.D., M.S.
Brigham and Women's Hospital
Boston, Massachusetts

Elliott Israel, M.D.
Brigham and Women's Hospital
Boston, Massachusetts

Meyer Kattan, M.D.
Mount Sinai Medical Center
New York, New York

Jerry A. Krishnan. M.D., Ph.D.
The Johns Hopkins School of Medicine
Baltimore, Maryland

James T. Li, M.D., Ph.D., F.A.A.A.A.I.
Mayo Clinic
Rochester, Minnesota

Dennis R. Ownby, M.D.
Medical College of Georgia
Augusta, Georgia

Gary S. Rachelefsky, M.D.
University of California–Los Angeles, School of Medicine
Los Angeles, California

Brian H. Rowe, M.D., M.Sc., C.C.F.P. (E.M.), F.C.C.P.
University of Alberta Hospital
Edmonton, Alberta, Canada

E. Rand Sutherland, M.D., M.P.H.
National Jewish Medical and Research Center
Denver, Colorado

Sandra R. Wilson, Ph.D.
Palo Alto Medical Foundation
Palo Alto, California

Robert A. Wood, M.D.
The Johns Hopkins School of Medicine
Baltimore, Maryland

Robert Zeiger, M.D.
Kaiser Permanente Medical Center
San Diego, California

Dr. Apter owns stock in Johnson & Johnson. She has received funding/grant support for research projects from the NHLBI.

Dr. Clark has no relevant financial interest.

Dr. Fulhlbrigge has served on the Speakers' Bureau of GlaxoSmithKline, the Advisory Boards of GlaxoSmithKline and Merck, the Data Systems Monitoring Board for a clinical trial sponsored by Sepracor, and as a consultant for GlaxoSmithKline. She has received honoraria from GlaxoSmithKline and Merck, and funding/grant support for a research project from Boehringer Ingelheim.

Dr. Israel has served on the Speakers' Bureau of Genentech and Merck, and as a consultant for Asthmatx, Critical Therapeutics, Genentech, Merck, Novartis Pharmaceuticals, Protein Design Labs, Schering-Plough Company, and Wyeth. He has received funding/grant support for research projects from Asthmatx, Boehringer Ingelheim, Centocor, Genentech, GlaxoSmithKline, and Merck.

Dr. Kattan has served on the Speakers' Bureau of AstraZeneca.

Dr. Krishnan has received funding/grant support for a research project from Hill-Rom, Inc.

Dr. Li has received funding/grant support for research projects from the American Lung Association, GlaxoSmithKline, Pharming, and ZLB Behring.

Dr. Ownby has no relevant financial interest.

Dr. Rachelefsky has served on the Speakers' Bureaus of AstraZeneca, GlaxoSmithKline, IVAX, Medpointe, Merck, and Schering Plough. He has received honoraria from AstraZeneca, GlaxoSmithKline, IVAX, Medpointe, Merck, and Schering Plough.

Dr. Rowe has served on the Advisory Boards of Abbott, AstraZeneca, Boehringer Ingelheim, and GlaxoSmithKline. He has received honoraria from Abbott, AstraZeneca, Boehringer Ingelheim, and GlaxoSmithKline. He has received funding/grant support for research projects from Abbott, AstraZeneca, Boehringer Ingelheim, GlaxoSmith-Kline, and Trudell.

Dr. Sutherland has served on the Speakers' Bureau of Novartis/Genentech and the Advisory Board of Dey Laboratories. He has received honoraria from IVAX and funding/grant support for research projects from GlaxoSmithKline and the NIH.

Dr. Wilson has served as a consultant for the Department of Urology, University of California, San Francisco (UCSF); Asthmatx, Inc.; and the Stanford UCSF Evidence-Based Practice Center. She has received funding/grant support for research projects from the NHLBI and from a subcontract to Stanford University from Blue Shield Foundation.

Dr. Wood has served on the Speakers' Bureaus of Dey Laboratories, GlaxoSmithKline, and Merck; on the Advisory Board of Dey Laboratories; and as a consultant to Dey Laboratories. He has received honoraria from Dey Laboratories, GlaxoSmithKline, and Merck, and funding/grant support for a research project from Genentech.

Dr. Zeiger has served on the Data Monitoring Board of Genentech, Advisory Board of GlaxoSmithKline, and as a consultant for Aerocrine, AstraZeneca, and Genentech. He has received honoraria from AstraZeneca and funding/grant support for a research project from Sanofi-Aventis.

National Heart, Lung, and Blood Institute

Robinson (Rob) Fulwood, Ph.D., M.S.P.H.
Branch Chief, Enhanced Dissemination and
    Utilization Branch
Division for the Application of Research Discoveries

James P. Kiley, Ph.D.
Director
Division of Lung Diseases

Gregory J. Morosco, Ph.D., M.P.H.
Associate Director for Prevention, Education, and
    Control
Director
Division for the Application of Research Discoveries

Diana K. Schmidt, M.P.H.
Coordinator
National Asthma Education and Prevention Program

Virginia S. Taggart, M.P.H.
Program Director
Division of Lung Diseases

American Institutes for Research

Heather Banks, M.A., M.A.T.
Senior Editor

Patti Louthian
Senior Desktop Publisher

Karen L. Soeken, Ph.D.
Methodologist

Mary Tierney, M.D.
Project Manager

Preface

The Expert Panel Report 3 (EPR—3) Summary Report 2007: Guidelines for the Diagnosis and Management of Asthma was developed by an expert panel commissioned by the National Asthma Education and Prevention Program (NAEPP) Coordinating Committee (CC), coordinated by the National Heart, Lung, and Blood Institute (NHLBI) of the National Institutes of Health.

Using the 1997 EPR—2 guidelines and the 2002 update on selected topics as the framework, the expert panel organized the literature review and updated recommendations for managing asthma long term and for managing exacerbations around four essential components of asthma care, namely: assessment and monitoring, patient education, control of factors contributing to asthma severity, and pharmacologic treatment. Subtopics were developed for each of these four broad categories.

The EPR—3 Full Report and the EPR—3 Summary Report 2007 have been developed under the excellent leadership of Dr. William Busse, Panel Chair. The NHLBI is grateful for the tremendous dedication of time and outstanding work of all the members of the expert panel, and for the advice from an expert consultant group in developing this report. Sincere appreciation is also extended to the NAEPP CC and the Guidelines Implementation Panel as well as other stakeholder groups (professional societies, voluntary health, government, consumer/patient advocacy organizations, and industry) for their invaluable comments during the public review period that helped to enhance the scientific credibility and practical utility of this document.

Ultimately, the broad change in clinical practice depends on the influence of local primary care physicians and other health professionals who not only provide state-of-the-art care to their patients, but also communicate to their peers the importance of doing the same. The NHLBI and its partners will forge new initiatives based on these guidelines to stimulate adoption of the recommendations at all levels, but particularly with primary care clinicians at the community level. We ask for the assistance of every reader in reaching our ultimate goal: improving asthma care and the quality of life for every asthma patient with asthma

Gregory Morosco, Ph.D., M.P.H.
Director
Division for the Application of Research Discoveries
National Heart, Lung, and Blood Institute

James Kiley, Ph.D.
Director
Division of Lung Diseases
National Heart, Lung, and Blood Institute

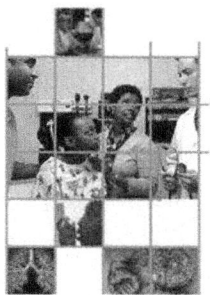

Introduction

More than 22 million Americans have asthma, and it is one of the most common chronic diseases of childhood, affecting an estimated 6 million children. The burden of asthma affects the patients, their families, and society in terms of lost work and school, lessened quality of life, and avoidable emergency department (ED) visits, hospitalizations, and deaths. Improved scientific understanding of asthma has led to significant improvements in asthma care, and the National Asthma Education and Prevention Program (NAEPP) has been dedicated to translating these research findings into clinical practice through publication and dissemination of clinical practice guidelines. The first NAEPP guidelines were published in 1991, and updates were made in 1997, 2002, and now with the current report. Important gains have been made in reducing morbidity and mortality rates due to asthma; however, challenges remain. The NAEPP hopes that the "Expert Panel Report 3: Guidelines for the Diagnosis and Management of Asthma—Full Report 2007" (EPR—3: Full Report 2007) will support the efforts of those who already incorporate best practices and will help enlist even greater numbers of primary care clinicians, asthma specialists, health care systems and providers, and communities to join together in making quality asthma care available to all people who have asthma. The goal, simply stated, is to help people with asthma control their asthma so that they can be active all day and sleep well at night.

This EPR—3: Summary Report 2007 presents the key recommendations from the EPR—3: Full Report 2007 (See www.nhlbi.nih.gov/guidelines/asthma/asthgdln.htm). Detailed recommendations, the levels of scientific evidence upon which they are based, citations from the published scientific literature, discussion of the Expert Panel's rationale for the recommendations, and description of methods used to develop the report are included in that resource document. Because EPR—3: Full Report 2007 is an update of previous NAEPP guidelines, highlights of major changes in the update are presented below, and figure 1 presents a summary of recommended key clinical activities.

HIGHLIGHTS OF MAJOR CHANGES IN EPR—3: FULL REPORT 2007

The following are highlights of major changes. Many recommendations were updated or expanded based on new evidence. See EPR—3: Full Report 2007 for key differences at the beginning of each section and for a full discussion.

New focus on monitoring asthma control as the goal for asthma therapy and distinguishing between classifying asthma severity and monitoring asthma control.
- Severity: the intrinsic intensity of the disease process. Assess asthma severity to initiate therapy.
- Control: the degree to which the manifestations of asthma are minimized by therapeutic interventions and the goals of therapy are met. Assess and monitor asthma control to adjust therapy.

New focus on impairment and risk as the two key domains of severity and control, and multiple measures for assessment. The domains represent different manifestations of asthma, they may not correlate with each other, and they may respond differentially to treatment.
- Impairment: frequency and intensity of symptoms and functional limitations the patient is experiencing currently or has recently experienced.
- Risk: the likelihood of either asthma exacerbations, progressive decline in lung function (or, for children, lung growth), or risk of adverse effects from medication.

Modifications in the stepwise approach to managing asthma long term.
- Treatment recommendations are presented for three age groups (0–4 years of age, 5–11 years of age, and youths ≥12 years of age and adults). The course of the disease may change over time; the relevance of different measures of impairment or risk and the potential short- and long-term impact of medications may be age related; and varied levels of scientific evidence are available for these three age groups.
- The stepwise approach expands to six steps to simplify the actions within each step. Previous guidelines had several progressive actions within different steps; these are now separated into different steps.
- Medications have been repositioned within the six steps of care.
  - Inhaled corticosteroids (ICSs) continue as preferred long-term control therapy for all ages.
  - Combination of long-acting beta$_2$-agonist (LABA) and ICS is presented as an equally preferred option, with increasing the dose of ICS in step 3 care, in patients 5 years of age or older. This approach balances the established beneficial effects of combination therapy in older children and adults with the increased risk for severe exacerbations, although uncommon, associated with daily use of LABA.
  - Omalizumab is recommended for consideration for youths ≥12 years of age who have allergies or for adults who require step 5 or 6 care (severe asthma). Clinicians who administer omalizumab should be prepared and equipped to identify and treat anaphylaxis that may occur.

New emphasis on multifaceted approaches to patient education and to the control of environmental factors or comorbid conditions that affect asthma.
- Patient education for a partnership is encouraged in expanded settings.
  - Patient education should occur at all points of care: clinic settings (offering separate self-management programs as well as integrating education into every patient visit), Emergency Departments (EDs) and hospitals, pharmacies, schools and other community settings, and patients' homes.
  - Provider education should encourage clinician and health care systems support of the partnership (e.g., through interactive continuing medical education, communication skills training, clinical pathways, and information system supports for clinical decisionmaking.
- Environmental control includes several strategies:
  - Multifaceted approaches to reduce exposures are necessary; single interventions are generally ineffective.
  - Consideration of subcutaneous immunotherapy for patients who have allergies at steps 2–4 of care (mild or moderate persistent asthma) when there is a clear relationship between symptoms and exposure to an allergen to which the patient is sensitive. Clinicians should be prepared to treat anaphylaxis that may occur.
  - Potential benefits to asthma control by treating comorbid conditions that affect asthma.

Modifications to treatment strategies for managing asthma exacerbations. These changes:
- Simplify the classification of severity of exacerbations. For the urgent or emergency care setting: <40 percent predicted forced expiratory volume in 1 second (FEV_1) or peak expiratory flow (PEF) indicates severe exacerbation and potential benefit from use of adjunctive therapies; ≥70 percent predicted FEV_1 or PEF is a goal for discharge from the emergency care setting.
- Encourage development of prehospital protocols for emergency medical services to allow administration of albuterol, oxygen, and, with medical oversight, anticholinergics and oral systemic corticosteroids.
- Modify recommendations on medications:
  - Add levalbuterol.
  - Add magnesium sulfate or heliox for severe exacerbations unresponsive to initial treatments.
  - Emphasize use of oral corticosteroids. Doubling the dose of ICS for home management is not effective.
  - Emphasize that anticholinergics are used in emergency care, not hospital care.
  - Add consideration of initiating ICS at discharge.

Figure 1. SUMMARY OF RECOMMENDED KEY CLINICAL ACTIVITIES FOR THE DIAGNOSIS AND MANAGEMENT OF ASTHMA

Clinical Issue	Key Clinical Activities	Action Steps
DIAGNOSIS		
	Establish asthma diagnosis.	Use medical history and physical examination to determine that symptoms of recurrent episodes of airflow obstruction are present.
		Use spirometry in all patients ≥5 years of age to determine that airway obstruction is at least partially reversible.
		Consider alternative causes of airway obstruction.
MANAGING ASTHMA LONG TERM	Goal of asthma therapy is asthma control: ■ Reduce impairment (prevent chronic symptoms, require infrequent use of short-acting beta$_2$-agonist (SABA), maintain (near) normal lung function and normal activity levels). ■ Reduce risk (prevent exacerbations, minimize need for emergency care or hospitalization, prevent loss of lung function, or for children, prevent reduced lung growth, have minimal or no adverse effects of therapy).	
Four Components of Care		
Assessment and Monitoring	Assess asthma severity to initiate therapy.	Use severity classification chart, assessing both domains of impairment and risk, to determine initial treatment.
	Assess asthma control to monitor and adjust therapy.	Use asthma control chart, assessing both domains of impairment and risk, to determine if therapy should be maintained or adjusted (step up if necessary, step down if possible).
		Use multiple measures of impairment and risk: different measures assess different manifestations of asthma; they may not correlate with each other; and they may respond differently to therapy. Obtain lung function measures by spirometry at least every 1–2 years, more frequently for not-well-controlled asthma.
	Schedule followup care.	Asthma is highly variable over time, and periodic monitoring is essential. In general, consider scheduling patients at 2- to 6-week intervals while gaining control; at 1–6 month intervals, depending on step of care required or duration of control, to monitor if sufficient control is maintained; at 3-month intervals if a step down in therapy is anticipated.
		Assess asthma control, medication technique, written asthma action plan, patient adherence and concerns at every visit.
Education	Provide self-management education.	Teach and reinforce: ■ Self-monitoring to assess level of asthma control and signs of worsening asthma (either symptom or peak flow monitoring shows similar benefits for most patients). Peak flow monitoring may be particularly helpful for patients who have difficulty perceiving symptoms, a history of severe exacerbations, or moderate or severe asthma. ■ Using written asthma action plan (review differences between long-term control and quick-relief medication). ■ Taking medication correctly (inhaler technique and use of devices). ■ Avoiding environmental factors that worsen asthma. Tailor education to literacy level of patient. Appreciate the potential role of a patient's cultural beliefs and practices in asthma management.

Figure 1. SUMMARY OF RECOMMENDED KEY CLINICAL ACTIVITIES FOR THE DIAGNOSIS AND MANAGEMENT OF ASTHMA (continued)

Clinical Issue	Key Clinical Activities	Action Steps
Four Components of Care (continued)		
Education (continued)	Develop a written asthma action plan in partnership with patient. Integrate education into all points of care where health professionals interact with patients.	Agree on treatment goals and address patient concerns.
		Provide instructions for (1) daily management (long-term control medication, if appropriate, and environmental control measures) and (2) managing worsening asthma (how to adjust medication, and know when to seek medical care).
		Involve all members of the health care team in providing/reinforcing education, including physicians, nurses, pharmacists, respiratory therapists, and asthma educators.
		Encourage education at all points of care: clinics (offering separate self-management education programs as well as incorporating education into every patient visit), Emergency Departments and hospitals, pharmacies, schools and other community settings, and patients' homes.
		Use a variety of educational strategies and methods.
Control Environmental Factors and Comorbid conditions	Recommend measures to control exposures to allergens and pollutants or irritants that make and asthma worse.	Determine exposures, history of symptoms in presence of exposures, and sensitivities (In patients who have persistent asthma, use skin or in vitro testing to assess sensitivity to perennial indoor allergens.).
		Advise patients on ways to reduce exposure to those allergens and pollutants, or irritants to which the patient is sensitive. Multifaceted approaches are beneficial; single steps alone are generally ineffective. Advise all patients and pregnant women to avoid exposure to tobacco smoke.
		Consider allergen immunotherapy, by specifically trained personnel, for patients who have persistent asthma and when there is clear evidence of a relationship between symptoms and exposure to an allergen to which the patient is sensitive.
	Treat comorbid conditions.	Consider especially: allergic bronchopulmonary aspergillosis; gastroesophageal reflux, obesity, obstructive sleep apnea, rhinitis and sinusitis, and stress or depression. Recognition and treatment of these conditions may improve asthma control.
		Consider inactivated influenza vaccine for all patients over 6 months of age.
Medications	Select medication and delivery devices to meet patient's needs and circumstances.	Use stepwise approach (See below.) to identify appropriate treatment options.
		Inhaled corticosteroids (ICSs) are the most effective long-term control therapy. When choosing among treatment options, consider domain of relevance to the patient (impairment, risk, or both), patient's history of response to the medication, and patient's willingness and ability to use the medication.

Figure 1. SUMMARY OF RECOMMENDED KEY CLINICAL ACTIVITIES FOR THE DIAGNOSIS AND MANAGEMENT OF ASTHMA (continued)

Clinical Issue	Key Clinical Activities	Action Steps
Stepwise Approach		
General Principles for All Age Groups	Incorporate four components of care.	Include medications, patient education, environmental control measures, and management of comorbidities at each step. Monitor asthma control regularly (See above, assessment and monitoring.).
	Initiate therapy based on asthma severity.	For patients not taking long-term control therapy, select treatment step based on severity (See figures on stepwise approach for different age groups.). Patients who have persistent asthma require daily long-term control medication.
	Adjust therapy based on asthma control.	Once therapy is initiated, monitor the level of asthma control and adjust therapy accordingly: step up if necessary and step down if possible to identify the minimum amount of medication required to maintain asthma control.
		Refer to an asthma specialist for consultation or comanagment if there are difficulties achieving or maintaining control; step 4 care or higher is required (step 3 care or higher for children 0–4 years of age); immunotherapy or omalizumab is considered; or additional testing is indicated; or if the patient required 2 bursts of oral systemic corticosticosteroids in the past year or a hospitalization.
Ages 0–4 Years	Consider daily long-term control therapy.	Young children may be at high risk for severe exacerbations, yet have low levels of impairment between exacerbations. Initiate daily long-term control therapy for:
		■ Children who had ≥4 episodes of wheezing the past year that lasted >1 day and affected sleep AND who have a positive asthma risk profile, either (1) one of the following: parental history of asthma, physician diagnosis of atopic dermatitis, or evidence of sensitization to aeroallergens OR (2) two of the following: sensitization to foods, ≥4 percent blood eosinophilia, or wheezing apart from colds.
		Consider initiating daily long-term control therapy for:
		■ Children who consistently require SABA treatment >2 days per week for >4 weeks.
		■ Children who have two exacerbations requiring oral systemic corticosteroids within 6 months.
	Monitor response closely, and adjust treatment.	If no clear and positive response occurs within 4–6 weeks and the patient's/caregiver's medication technique and adherence are satisfactory, stop the treatment and consider alternative therapies or diagnoses.
		If clear benefit is sustained for at least 3 months, consider step down to evaluate the continued need for daily therapy. Children this age have high rates of spontaneous remission of symptoms.

Figure 1. SUMMARY OF RECOMMENDED KEY CLINICAL ACTIVITIES FOR THE DIAGNOSIS AND MANAGEMENT OF ASTHMA (continued)

Clinical Issue	Key Clinical Activities	Action Steps
Stepwise Approach (continued)		
Ages 5–11 Years	Involve child in developing a written asthma action plan.	Address child's concerns, preferences, and school schedule in selecting treatments.
		Encourage students to take a copy of written asthma action plan to school/afterschool activities.
	Promote physical activity.	Treat exercise-induced bronchospasm (EIB) (See below.) Step up daily therapy if the child has poor endurance or symptoms during normal play activities.
	Monitor for disease progression and loss of lung growth.	Treatment will not alter underlying progression of the disease, but a step up in therapy may be required to maintain asthma control.
Ages 12 and Older	Involve youths in developing written asthma action plan.	Address youth's concerns, preferences, and school schedule in selecting treatment.
		Encourage students to take a copy of written asthma action plan to school/afterschool activities.
	Promote physical activity.	Treat EIB. Step up daily therapy if the child has poor endurance or symptoms during normal daily activities.
	Assess possible benefit of treatment in older patients.	Establish reversibility with a short course of oral systemic corticosteroids.
	Adjust medications to address coexisting medical conditions common among older patients.	Consider, for example: calcium and vitamin D supplements for patients who take ICS and have risk factors for osteoporosis; increased sensitivity to side effects of bronchodilators with increasing age; increased drug interactions with theophylline; medications for arthritis (NSAIDs), hypertension, or glaucoma (beta blockers) may exacerbate asthma.
Exercise-Induced Bronchospasm (EIB)	Prevent EIB	Treatment strategies to prevent EIB include: ■ Long-term control therapy. ■ Pretreatment before exercise with SABA, leukotriene receptor antagonists (LTRAs), cromolyn or nedocromil; frequent or chronic use of long acting beta$_2$-agonist (LABA) for pretreatment is discouraged, as it may disguise poorly controlled persistent asthma. ■ Warmup period or a mask or scarf over the mouth for cold-induced EIB.
Pregnancy	Maintain asthma control through pregnancy.	Monitor asthma control during all prenatal visits; asthma worsens in one-third of women during pregnancy and improves in one-third; medications should be adjusted accordingly.
		It is safer to be treated with asthma medications than to have poorly controlled asthma. Maintaining lung function is important to ensure oxygen supply to the fetus.
		Albuterol is the preferred SABA. ICS is the preferred long-term control medication (Budesonide is preferred because more data are available on this medication during pregnancy.).
Surgery	Reduce risks for complications during and after surgery.	Assess asthma control prior to surgery. If lung function is not well controlled, provide medications to improve lung function. A short course of oral systemic corticosteroids may be necessary.
		For patients receiving oral systemic corticosteroids during 6 months prior to surgery, and for selected patients on high dose ICS, give 100 mg hydrocortisone every 8 hours intravenously during the surgical period, and reduce the dose rapidly within 24 hours after surgery.

Figure 1. SUMMARY OF RECOMMENDED KEY CLINICAL ACTIVITIES FOR THE DIAGNOSIS AND MANAGEMENT OF ASTHMA (continued)

Clinical Issue	Key Clinical Activities	Action Steps
Managing Exacerbations		
Home Management	Incorporate four components of care.	Include assessment and monitoring, patient education, environmental control, and medications.
	Develop a written asthma action plan.	Instruct patients how to: • Recognize early signs, symptoms, peak expiratory flow (PEF) measures that indicate worsening asthma. • Adjust medications (increase SABA and, in some cases, add oral systemic corticosteroids) and remove or withdraw from environmental factors contributing to the exacerbation. • Monitor response and seek medical care if there is serious deterioration or lack of response to treatment.

Management in the Urgent or Emergency Care Setting	Assess severity.
	Treat to relieve hypoxemia and airflow obstruction; reduce airway inflammation.
	Monitor response.
	Discharge with medication and patient education
		Treatment strategies include:
		• Assessing initial severity by lung function measures (for ages ≥5 years) and symptom and functional assessment
		• Supplemental oxygen
		• Repetitive or continuous SABA
		• Oral systemic corticosteroids
		• Monitoring response with serial assessment of lung function measures, pulse oximetry, and symptoms
		• Considering adjunctive treatments magnesium sulfate or heliox in severe exacerbations (e.g., forced expiratory volume in 1 second (FEV_1) or PEF <40 percent predicted) unresponsive to initial treatment
		• Providing at discharge:
		  — Medications: SABA, oral systemic corticosteroids; consider initiating ICS
		  — Referral to followup care
		  — An emergency department asthma discharge plan
		  — Review of inhaler technique and, whenever possible, environmental control measures

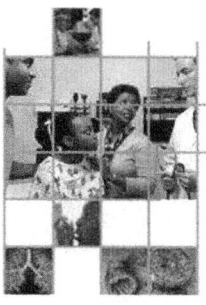

Asthma Definition and Implications for Treatment

Definition and Pathophysiology

Asthma is a complex disorder characterized by variable and recurring symptoms, airflow obstruction, bronchial hyperresponsiveness, and an underlying inflammation. The interaction of these features determines the clinical manifestations and severity of asthma (See figure 2, "The Interplay and Interaction Between Airway Inflammation and the Clinical Symptoms and Pathophysiology of Asthma.") and the response to treatment. The working definition of asthma is as follows:

Asthma is a chronic inflammatory disorder of the airways in which many cells and cellular elements play a role: in particular, mast cells, eosinophils, neutrophils (especially in sudden onset, fatal exacerbations, occupational asthma, and patients who smoke), T lymphocytes, macrophages, and epithelial cells. In susceptible individuals, this inflammation causes recurrent episodes of coughing (particularly at night or early in the morning), wheezing, breathlessness, and chest tightness. These episodes are usually associated with widespread but variable airflow obstruction that is often reversible either spontaneously or with treatment.

Airflow limitation is caused by a variety of changes in the airway, all in influenced by airway inflamation:

- Bronchoconstriction—bronchial smooth muscle contraction that quickly narrows the airways in response to exposure to a variety of stimuli, including allergens or irritants.
- Airway hyperresponsiveness—an exaggerated bronchoconstrictor response to stimuli.
- Airway edema—as the disease becomes more persistent and inflammation becomes more progressive, edema, mucus hypersecretion, and formation of inspissated mucus plugs further limit airflow.

Remodeling of airways may occur. Reversibility of airflow limitation may be incomplete in some patients. Persistent changes in airway structure occur, including sub-basement fibrosis, mucus hypersecretion, injury to epithelial cells, smooth muscle hypertrophy, and angiogenesis.

Recent studies provide insights on different phenotypes of asthma that exist. Different manifestations of asthma may have specific and varying patterns of inflammation (e.g., varying intensity, cellular mediator pattern, and therapeutic response). Further studies will determine if different treatment approaches benefit the different patterns of inflammation.

Figure 2. THE INTERPLAY AND INTERACTION BETWEEN AIRWAY INFLAMMATION AND THE CLINICAL SYMPTOMS AND PATHOPHYSIOLOGY OF ASTHMA

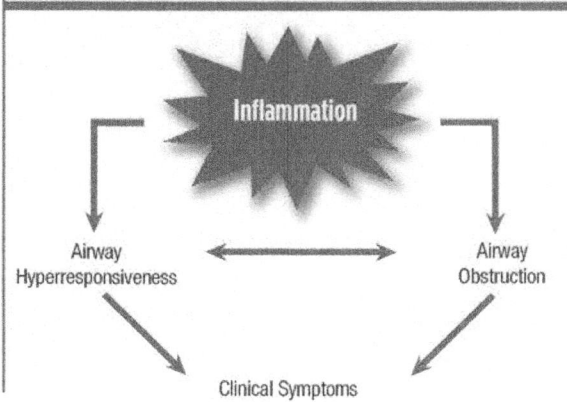

Causes of Asthma

The development of asthma appears to involve the interplay between host factors (particularly genetics) and environmental exposures that occur at a crucial time in the development of the immune system. A definitive cause of the inflammatory process leading to asthma has not yet been established.

- Innate immunity. Numerous factors may affect the balance between Th1-type and Th2- type cytokine responses in early life and increase the likelihood that the immune response will downregulate the Th1 immune response that fights infection and instead will be dominated by Th2 cells, leading to the expression of allergic diseases and asthma. This is known as the "hygiene hypothesis," which postulates that certain infections early in life, exposure to other children (e.g., presence of older siblings and early enrollment in childcare, which have greater likelihood of exposure to respiratory infection), less frequent use of antibiotics, and "country living" is associated with a Th1 response and lower incidence of asthma, whereas the absence of these factors is associated with a persistent Th2 response and higher rates of asthma. Interventions to prevent the onset of this process (e.g., with probiotics) are under study, but no recommendations can yet be made.

- Genetics. Asthma has an inheritable component, but the genetics involved remain complex. As the linkage of genetic factors to different asthma phenotypes becomes clearer, treatment approaches may become directed to specific patient phenotypes and genotypes.

- Environmental factors.
  — Two major factors are the most important in the development, persistence, and possibly the severity of asthma: airborne allergens (particularly sensitization and exposure to house-dust mite and Alternaria) and viral respiratory infections (including respiratory syncytial virus [RSV] and rhinovirus).

  — Other environmental factors are under study: tobacco smoke (exposure in utero is associated with an increased risk of wheezing, but it is not certain this is linked to subsequent development of asthma), air pollution (ozone and particular matter) and diet (obesity or low intake of antioxidants and omega-3 fatty acids). The association of these factors with the onset of asthma has not been clearly defined. A number of clinical trials have investigated dietary and environmental manipulations, but these trials have not been sufficiently long term or conclusive to permit recommendations.

Implications for Treatment

Knowledge of the importance of inflammation to the central features of asthma continues to expand and underscores inflammation as a primary target of treatment. Studies indicate that current therapeutic approaches are effective in controlling symptoms, reducing airflow limitation, and preventing exacerbations, but currently available treatments do not appear to prevent the progression of asthma in children. As various phenotypes of asthma are defined and inflammatory and genetic factors become more apparent, new therapeutic approaches may be developed that will allow even greater specificity to tailor treatment to the individual patient's needs and circumstances.

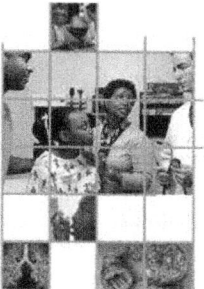

Diagnosis of Asthma

To establish a diagnosis of asthma, the clinician should determine that symptoms of recurrent episodes of airflow obstruction or airway hyperresponsiveness are present; airflow obstruction is at least partially reversible; and alternative diagnoses are excluded.

KEY SYMPTOM INDICATORS FOR CONSIDERING A DIAGNOSIS OF ASTHMA

The presence of multiple key indicators increases the probability of asthma, but spirometry is needed to establish a diagnosis.

- Wheezing—high-pitched whistling sounds when breathing out—especially in children. A lack of wheezing and a normal chest examination do not exclude asthma.
- History of any of the following:
  - Cough (worse particularly at night)
  - Recurrent wheeze
  - Recurrent difficulty in breathing
  - Recurrent chest tightness
- Symptoms occur or worsen in the presence of:
  - Exercise
  - Viral infection
  - Inhalant allergens (e.g., animals with fur or hair, house-dust mites, mold, pollen)
  - Irritants (tobacco or wood smoke, airborne chemicals)
  - Changes in weather
  - Strong emotional expression (laughing or crying hard)
  - Stress
  - Menstrual cycles
- Symptoms occur or worsen at night, awakening the patient.

- Episodic symptoms of airflow obstruction or airway hyperresponsiveness are present.
- Airflow obstruction is at least partially reversible, measured by spirometry. Reversibility is determined by an increase in FEV_1 of >200 mL and ≥12 percent from baseline measure after inhalation of short-acting beta$_2$-agonist (SABA). Some studies indicate that an increase of ≥10 percent of the predicted FEV_1 after inhalation of a SABA may have higher likelihood of separating patients who have asthma from those who have chronic obstructive pulmonary disease (COPD).
- Alternative diagnoses are excluded. See discussion below.

Recommended methods to establish the diagnosis are:

- **Detailed medical history.** See figure 3, "Suggested Items for Medical History," for questions to include.
- **Physical examination** may reveal findings that increase the probability of asthma, but the absence of these findings does not rule out asthma, because the disease is variable and signs may be absent between episodes. The examination focuses on:
  - upper respiratory tract (increased nasal secretion, mucosal swelling, and/or nasal polyp;
  - chest (sounds of wheezing during normal breathing or prolonged phase of forced exhalation, hyperexpansion of the thorax, use of accessory muscles, appearance of hunched shoulders, chest deformity); and
  - skin (atopic dermatitis, eczema).
- **Spirometry** can demonstrate obstruction and assess reversibility in patients ≥5 years of age. Patients' perceptions of airflow obstruction are highly variable. Spirometry is an essential objective measure to establish the diagnosis of asthma,

DIFFERENTIAL DIAGNOSTIC POSSIBILITIES FOR ASTHMA

Infants and Children

Upper airway diseases
- Allergic rhinitis and sinusitis

Obstructions involving large airways
- Foreign body in trachea or bronchus
- Vocal cord dysfunction (VCD)
- Vascular rings or laryngeal webs
- Laryngotracheomalacia, tracheal stenosis, or bronchostenosis
- Enlarged lymph nodes or tumor

Obstructions involving small airways
- Viral bronchiolitis or obliterative bronchiolitis
- Cystic fibrosis
- Bronchopulmonary dysplasia
- Heart disease

Other causes
- Recurrent cough not due to asthma
- Aspiration from swallowing mechanism dysfunction or gastroesophageal reflux

Adults
- Chronic obstructive pulmonary disease (COPD) (e.g., chronic bronchitis or emphysema)
- Congestive heart failure
- Pulmonary embolism
- Mechanical obstruction of the airways (benign and malignant tumors)
- Pulmonary infiltration with eosinophilia
- Cough secondary to drugs (e.g., angiotensin-converting enzyme [ACE] inhibitors)
- Vocal cord dysfunction (VCD)

---

because the medical history and physical examination are not reliable means of excluding other diagnoses or of assessing lung status. Spirometry is generally recommended, rather than measurements by a peak flow meter, due to wide variability in peak flow meters and reference values. Peak flow meters are designed for monitoring, not as diagnostic tools.

A differential diagnosis of asthma should be considered. Recurrent episodes of cough and wheezing most often are due to asthma in both children and adults; however, other significant causes of airway obstruction leading to wheeze must be considered both in the initial diagnosis and if there is no clear response to initial therapy.

- **Additional studies are not routinely necessary but may be useful when considering alternative diagnoses.**

  — **Additional pulmonary function studies** will help if there are questions about COPD (diffusing capacity), a restrictive defect (measures of lung volumes), or VCD (evaluation of inspiratory flow-volume loops).

  — **Bronchoprovocation** with methacholine, histamine, cold air, or exercise challenge may be useful when asthma is suspected and spirometry is normal or near normal. For safety reasons, bronchoprovocation should be carried out only by a trained individual. A positive test is diagnostic for airway hyperresponsiveness, which is a characteristic feature of asthma but can also be present in other conditions. Thus, a positive test is consistent with asthma, but a negative test may be more helpful to rule out asthma.

  — **Chest x ray** may be needed to exclude other diagnoses.

  — **Biomarkers of inflammation** are currently being evaluated for their usefulness in the diagnosis and assessment of asthma. Biomarkers include total and differential cell count and mediator assays in sputum, blood, urine, and exhaled air.

- **Common diagnostic challenges include the following:**

  — **Cough variant asthma.** Cough can be the principal—or only—manifestation of asthma, especially in young children.

FIGURE 3. SUGGESTED ITEMS FOR MEDICAL HISTORY*

A detailed medical history of the new patient who is known or thought to have asthma should address the following items

1. **Symptoms**
   Cough
   Wheezing
   Shortness of breath
   Chest tightness
   Sputum production

2. **Pattern of symptoms**
   Perennial, seasonal, or both
   Continual, episodic, or both
   Onset, duration, frequency (number of days or nights, per week or month)
   Diurnal variations, especially nocturnal and on awakening in early morning

3. **Precipitating and/or aggravating factors**
   Viral respiratory infections
   Environmental allergens, indoor (e.g., mold, house-dust mite, cockroach, animal dander or secretory products) and outdoor (e.g., pollen)
   Characteristics of home including age, location, cooling and heating system, wood-burning stove, humidifier, carpeting over concrete, presence of molds or mildew, presence of pets with fur or hair, characteristics of rooms where patient spends time (e.g., bedroom and living room with attention to bedding, floor covering, stuffed furniture)
   Smoking (patient and others in home or daycare)
   Exercise
   Occupational chemicals or allergens
   Environmental change (e.g., moving to new home; going on vacation; and/or alterations in workplace, work processes, or materials used)
   Irritants (e.g., tobacco smoke, strong odors, air pollutants, occupational chemicals, dusts and particulates, vapors, gases, and aerosols)
   Emotions (e.g., fear, anger, frustration, hard crying or laughing)
   Stress (e.g., fear, anger, frustration)
   Drugs (e.g., aspirin; and other nonsteroidal anti-inflammatory drugs, beta-blockers including eye drops, others)
   Food, food additives, and preservatives (e.g., sulfites)
   Changes in weather, exposure to cold air
   Endocrine factors (e.g., menses, pregnancy, thyroid disease)
   Comorbid conditions (e.g. sinusitis, rhinitis, gastroesophageal reflux disease (GERD)

4. **Development of disease and treatment**
   Age of onset and diagnosis
   History of early-life injury to airways (e.g., bronchopulmonary dysplasia, pneumonia, parental smoking)
   Progression of disease (better or worse)
   Present management and response, including plans for managing exacerbations
   Frequency of using short-acting beta$_2$-agonist (SABA)
   Need for oral corticosteroids and frequency of use

5. **Family history**
   History of asthma, allergy, sinusitis, rhinitis, eczema, or nasal polyps in close relatives

6. **Social history**
   Daycare, workplace, and school characteristics that may interfere with adherence
   Social factors that interfere with adherence, such as substance abuse
   Social support/social networks
   Level of education completed
   Employment

7. **History of exacerbations**
   Usual prodromal signs and symptoms
   Rapidity of onset
   Duration
   Frequency
   Severity (need for urgent care, hospitalization, intensive care unit (ICU) admission.)
   Life-threatening exacerbations (e.g., intubation, intensive care unit admission)
   Number and severity of exacerbations in the past year.
   Usual patterns and management (what works?)

8. **Impact of asthma on patient and family**
   Episodes of unscheduled care (emergency department (ED), urgent care, hospitalization)
   Number of days missed from school/work
   Limitation of activity, especially sports and strenuous work
   History of nocturnal awakening
   Effect on growth, development, behavior, school or work performance, and lifestyle
   Impact on family routines, activities, or dynamics
   Economic impact

9. **Assessment of patient's and family's perceptions of disease**
   Patient's, parent's, and spouse's or partner's knowledge of asthma and belief in the chronicity of asthma and in the efficacy of treatment
   Patient's perception and beliefs regarding use and long-term effects of medications
   Ability of patient and parents, spouse, or partner to cope with disease
   Level of family support and patient's and parents', spouse's, or partner's capacity to recognize severity of an exacerbation
   Economic resources
   Sociocultural beliefs

* This list does not represent a standardized assessment or diagnostic instrument. The validity and reliability of this list have not been assessed.

Diagnosis of Asthma

Monitoring of PEF or bronchoprovocation may be helpful. Diagnosis is confirmed by a positive response to asthma medications.

— **VCD** can mimic asthma, but it is a distinct disorder. VCD may coexist with asthma. Asthma medications typically do little, if anything, to relieve VCD symptoms. Variable flattening of the inspiratory flow loop on spirometry is strongly suggestive of VCD. Diagnosis of VCD is from indirect or direct vocal cord visualization during an episode, during which the abnormal adduction can be documented. VCD should be considered in difficult-to-treat, atypical asthma patients and in elite athletes who have exercise-related breathlessness unresponsive to asthma medication.

— **Gastroesophageal reflux disease (GERD), obstructive sleep apnea (OSA), and allergic bronchopulmonary aspergillosis (ABPA)** may coexist with asthma and complicate diagnosis. See the section on "Comorbid Conditions," for further discussion.

— **Children ages 0–4 years.** Diagnosis in infants and young children is challenging and is complicated by the difficulty in obtaining objective measurements of lung function in this age group. Caution is needed to avoid giving young children inappropriate prolonged asthma therapy. However, it is important to avoid underdiagnosing asthma, and thereby missing the opportunity to treat a child, by using such labels as "wheezy bronchitis," "recurrent pneumonia," or "reactive airway disease" (RAD). The chronic airway inflammatory response and structural changes that are characteristic of asthma can develop in the preschool years, and appropriate asthma treatment will reduce morbidity.

- **Consider referral to an asthma specialist if signs and symptoms are atypical, if there are problems with a differential diagnosis, or if additional testing is indicated.**

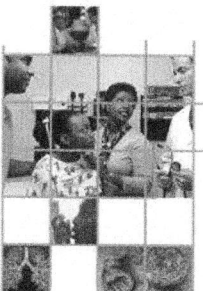

Managing Asthma Long Term

GOAL OF THERAPY: CONTROL OF ASTHMA

Reduce Impairment

- Prevent chronic and troublesome symptoms (e.g., coughing or breathlessness in the daytime, in the night, or after exertion).
- Require infrequent use (≤2 days a week) of inhaled SABA for quick relief of symptoms (not including prevention of exercise-induced bronchospasm [EIB]).
- Maintain (near) normal pulmonary function.
- Maintain normal activity levels (including exercise and other physical activity and attendance at school or work).
- Meet patients' and families' expectations of and satisfaction with asthma care.

Reduce Risk

- Prevent recurrent exacerbations of asthma and minimize the need for ED visits or hospitalizations.
- Prevent loss of lung function; for children, prevent reduced lung growth.
- Provide optimal pharmacotherapy with minimal or no adverse effects of therapy.

Achieving and maintaining asthma control requires four components of care: assessment and monitoring, education for a partnership in care, control of environmental factors and comorbid conditions that affect asthma, and medications. A stepwise approach to asthma management incorporates these four components, emphasizing that pharmacologic therapy is initiated based on asthma severity and adjusted (stepped up or down) based on the level of asthma control. Special considerations of therapeutic options within the stepwise approach may be necessary for situations such as exercise-induced bronchospasm (EIB), surgery, and pregnancy.

Four Components of Asthma Care

Component 1: Assessing and Monitoring Asthma Severity and Asthma Control

The functions of assessment and monitoring are closely linked to the concepts of severity, control, and responsiveness to treatment:

- **Severity:** the intrinsic intensity of the disease process. Severity is most easily and directly measured in a patient who is not receiving long-term control therapy. Severity can also be measured, once asthma control is achieved, by the step of care (i.e., the amount of medication) required to maintain control.

- **Control:** the degree to which the manifestations of asthma are minimized by therapeutic intervention and the goals of therapy are met.

- **Responsiveness:** the ease with which asthma control is achieved by therapy.

Asthma severity and asthma control include the domains of current impairment and future risk.

- **Impairment:** frequency and intensity of symptoms and functional limitations the patient is currently experiencing or has recently experienced.

- **Risk:** the likelihood of either asthma exacerbations, progressive decline in lung function (or, for children, reduced lung growth), or risk of adverse effects from medication.

This distinction emphasizes the multifaceted nature of asthma and the need to consider separately asthma's current, ongoing effects on the present quality of life and functional capacity and the future risk of adverse events. The two domains may respond differentially to treatment. For example, evidence demonstrates that some patients can have adequate control of symptoms and minimal day-to-day impairment, but still be at significant risk of exacerbations; these patients should be treated accordingly.

The specific measures used to assess severity and control are similar: symptoms, use of SABAs for quick relief of symptoms, limitations to normal activities due to asthma, pulmonary function, and exacerbations. Multiple measures are important, because different measures assess different manifestations of the disease and may not correlate with each other.

The concepts of severity and control are used as follows for managing asthma:

- **Assess severity to initiate therapy.** See section on "Stepwise Approach for Managing Asthma" for figures on classifying asthma severity and initiating therapy in different age groups. During a patient's initial presentation, if the patient is not currently taking long-term control medication, asthma severity is assessed to guide clinical decisions for initiating the appropriate medication and other therapeutic interventions.

- **Assess control to adjust therapy.** See section on "Stepwise Approach for Managing Asthma" for figures on assessing asthma control and adjusting therapy in different age groups. Once therapy is initiated, the emphasis for clinical management thereafter is changed to the assessment of asthma control. The level of asthma control will guide decisions either to maintain or to adjust therapy (i.e., step up if necessary, step down if possible).

- **For assessing a patient's overall asthma severity, once the most optimal asthma control is achieved and maintained,** or for population-based evaluations or clinical research, asthma severity can be inferred by correlating the level of severity with the lowest level of treatment required to maintain control.

Lowest level of treatment required to maintain control	Classification of Asthma Severity When Asthma Is Well Controlled			
		Persistent		
(See "Stepwise Approach for Managing Asthma" for treatment steps.)	Intermittent	Mild	Moderate	Severe
	Step 1	Step 2	Step 3 or Step 4	Step 5 or Step 6

However, the emphasis for clinical management is to assess asthma severity prior to initiating therapy and then to assess asthma control for monitoring and adjusting therapy.

For the initial assessment to characterize the patient's asthma and guide decisions for initiating therapy, use information from the diagnostic evaluation to:

- **Classify asthma severity.**

- **Identify precipitating factors** for episodic symptoms (e.g., exposure at home, work, daycare, or school to inhalant allergens or irritants).

- **Identify comorbid conditions** that may impede asthma management (e.g., sinusitis, rhinitis, GERD, OSA, obesity, stress, or depression).

- **Assess the patient's knowledge and skills** for self-management.

For periodic monitoring of asthma control to guide decisions for maintaining or adjusting therapy:

- **Instruct patients to monitor their asthma control in an ongoing manner. All patients should be taught how to recognize inadequate asthma control.**

  — Either symptom or peak flow monitoring is appropriate for most patients; evidence suggests the benefits are similar.

  — Consider daily peak-flow monitoring for patients who have moderate or severe persistent asthma, patients who have a history of severe exacerbations, and patients who poorly perceive airway obstruction or worsening asthma.

- **Monitor asthma control periodically in clinical visits,** because asthma is highly variable over time and therapy may need to be adjusted (stepped up if necessary, stepped down if possible). **The frequency of monitoring is a matter of clinical judgment. In general:**

FIGURE 4. SAMPLE PATIENT SELF-ASSESSMENT SHEET FOR FOLLOWUP VISITS*

Name:_____ Date:_____

Your Asthma Control

How many days in the past week have you had chest tightness, cough, shortness of breath, or wheezing (whistling in your chest)?

_____ 0 _____ 1 _____ 2 _____ 3 _____ 4 _____ 5 _____ 6 _____ 7

How many nights in the past week have you had chest tightness, cough, shortness of breath, or wheezing (whistling in your chest)?

_____ 0 _____ 1 _____ 2 _____ 3 _____ 4 _____ 5 _____ 6 _____ 7

Do you perform peak flow readings at home? _____ yes _____ no

If yes, did you bring your peak flow chart? _____ yes _____ no

How many days in the past week has asthma restricted your physical activity?

_____ 0 _____ 1 _____ 2 _____ 3 _____ 4 _____ 5 _____ 6 _____ 7

Have you had any asthma attacks since your last visit? _____ yes _____ no

Have you had any unscheduled visits to a doctor, including to the emergency department, since your last visit? _____ yes _____ no

How well controlled is your asthma, in your opinion?   ____ very well controlled
　　　　　　　　　　　　　　　　　　　　　　　　　　　　　　____ somewhat controlled
　　　　　　　　　　　　　　　　　　　　　　　　　　　　　　____ not well controlled

　　　　Average number of puffs per day of quick-relief
　　　　medication (short acting beta$_2$-agonist)　　　　　_____

Taking your medicine

What problems have you had taking your medicine or following your asthma action plan?

Please ask the doctor or nurse to review how you take your medicine.

Your questions

What questions or concerns would you like to discuss with the doctor?

How satisfied are you with your asthma care? ____ very satisfied
　　　　　　　　　　　　　　　　　　　　　　　____ somewhat satisfied
　　　　　　　　　　　　　　　　　　　　　　　____ not satisfied

*These questions are examples and do not represent a standardized assessment instrument. Other examples of asthma control questions: Asthma Control Questionnaire (Juniper); Asthma Therapy Assessment Questionnaire (Volmer); Asthma Control Test (Nathan); Asthma Control Score (Boulet)

- Schedule visits at 2- to 6-week intervals for patients who are just starting therapy or who require a step up in therapy to achieve or regain asthma control.
- Schedule visits at 1- to 6-month intervals, after asthma control is achieved, to monitor whether asthma control is maintained. The interval will depend on factors such as the duration of asthma control or the level of treatment required.
- Consider scheduling visits at 3-month intervals if a step down in therapy is anticipated.

■ **Assess asthma control, medication technique, the written asthma action plan, adherence, and patient concerns at every patient visit.** See figure 4 for a sample patient self-assessment of overall asthma control and asthma care.

■ Use spirometry to obtain objective measures of lung function.
- Perform spirometry at the following times:
  - At the initial assessment.
  - After treatment is initiated and symptoms and PEF have stabilized.
  - During periods of progressive or prolonged loss of asthma control.
  - At least every 1–2 years; more frequently depending on response to therapy.
- Low FEV_1 indicates current obstruction (impairment) and risk for future exacerbations (risk). For children, FEV_1/forced vital capacity (FVC) appears to be a more sensitive measure of severity and control in the impairment domain. FEV_1 is a useful measure of risk for exacerbations, although it is emphasized that even children who have normal lung function experience exacerbations.

■ **Minimally invasive markers** (called biomarkers) such as fractionated exhaled nitric oxide (FeNO) and sputum eosinophils may be useful, but bio markers require further evaluation before they can be recommended as clinical tools for routine management.

Component 2: Education for a Partnership in Care

A partnership between the clinician and the person who has asthma (and the caregiver, for children) is required for effective asthma management. By working together, an appropriate treatment can be selected, and the patient can learn self-management skills necessary to control asthma. Self-management education improves patient outcomes (e.g., reduced urgent care visits, hospitalizations, and limitations on activities as well as improved health status, quality of life, and perceived control of asthma) and can be cost-effective. Self-management education is an integral component of effective asthma care and should be treated as such by health care providers as well as by health care policies and reimbursements.

KEY EDUCATIONAL MESSAGES: TEACH AND REINFORCE AT EVERY OPPORTUNITY

Basic Facts About Asthma

- The contrast between airways of a person who has and a person who does not have asthma; the role of inflammation.
- What happens to the airways during an asthma attack.

Role of Medications: Understanding the Difference Between:

- Long-term control medications: prevent symptoms, often by reducing inflammation. Must be taken daily. Do not expect them to give quick relief.
- Quick-relief medications: SABAs relax airway muscles to provide prompt relief of symptoms. Do not expect them to provide long-term asthma control. Using SABA >2 days a week indicates the need for starting or increasing long-term control medications.

Patient Skills

- Taking medications correctly
  - Inhaler technique (demonstrate to the patient and have the patient return the demonstration).
  - Use of devices, as prescribed (e.g., valved holding chamber (VHC) or spacer, nebulizer).
- Identifying and avoiding environmental exposures that worsen the patient's asthma; e.g., allergens, irritants, tobacco smoke.
- Self-monitoring
  - Assess level of asthma control.
  - Monitor symptoms and, if prescribed, PEF measures.
  - Recognize early signs and symptoms of worsening asthma.
- Using a written asthma action plan to know when and how to:
  - Take daily actions to control asthma.
  - Adjust medication in response to signs of worsening asthma.
- Seeking medical care as appropriate.

Develop an active partnership with the patient and family by:

- Establishing open communications that consider cultural and ethnic factors, as well as language and health care literacy needs, of each patient and family.

- Identifying and addressing patient and family concerns about asthma and asthma treatment.

- Developing treatment goals and selecting medications together with the patient and family, allowing full participation in treatment decision making.

- Encouraging self-monitoring and self-management by reviewing at each opportunity the patient's reports of asthma symptoms and response to treatment.

Provide to all patients a written asthma action plan that includes instructions for both daily management (long-term control medication, if appropriate, and environmental control measures) and actions to manage worsening asthma (what signs, symptoms, and PEF measurements (if used) indicate worsening asthma; what medications to take in response; what signs and symptoms indicate the need for immediate medical care). Written asthma action plans are particularly recommended for patients who have moderate or severe persistent asthma (i.e., requiring treatment at step 4, 5, or 6), a history of severe exacerbations, or poorly controlled asthma. See figures 5 and 6 for samples of written asthma action plans.

Integrate asthma self-management education into all aspects of asthma care. Asthma self management requires repetition and reinforcement. It should:

- Begin at the time of diagnosis and continue through followup care. See figure 7, "Delivery of Asthma Education by Clinicians During Patient Care Visits," for a sample of how to incorporate teaching into routine clinic visits.

- Involve all members of the health care team, including physicians, nurses, pharmacists, respiratory therapists, and asthma educators, as well as other health professionals who come in contact with asthma patients and their families.

- Occur at all points of care where health care professionals interact with patients who have asthma. The strongest evidence supports self-management education in the clinic setting. Evidence also supports education provided in patients' homes, pharmacies, targeted education in EDs and hospitals, and selected programs in schools and other community sites. Proven community programs should be considered because of their potential to reach large numbers of people who have asthma and encourage "asthma-friendly" support from their families and community environments.

- Use a variety of educational strategies to reach people who have varying levels of health literacy or learning styles. Individual instruction, group programs, written materials (at a 5th grade reading level or below), video- or audiotapes, and computer and Internet programs all provide effective educational opportunities. See figure 8, "Asthma Education Resources," for a sample of available resources.

- Incorporate individualized case/care management by trained health care professionals for patients who have poorly controlled asthma and have recurrent visits to the emergency department or hospital. This will provide tailored self-management education and skills training.

Encourage patients' adherence to the written asthma action plan by:

- Choosing treatment that achieves outcomes and addresses preferences that are important to the patient, and reminding patients that adherence will help them achieve the outcomes they want.

- Reviewing with the patient at each visit the success of the treatment plan to achieve asthma control and make adjustments as needed.

- Reviewing patients' concerns about their asthma or treatment at every visit. Inquire about any difficulties encountered in adhering to the written asthma action plan.

- Assessing the patient's and family's level of social support, and encouraging family involvement.

- Tailoring the self-management approach to the needs and literacy levels of the patient, and maintaining sensitivity to cultural beliefs and ethnocultural practices.

Encourage health care provider and health care system support of the therapeutic partnership by:

- Incorporating effective clinician education strategies,

FIGURE 5. SAMPLE ASTHMA ACTION PLAN—ADULT

ENGLISH

My Asthma Action Plan

Patient Name: _____
Medical Record #: _____

Physician's Name: _____ DOB: _____

Physician's Phone #: _____ Completed by: _____ Date: _____

Long-Term-Control Medicines	How Much To Take	How Often	Other Instructions
		_____ times per day EVERY DAY!	
		_____ times per day EVERY DAY!	
		_____ times per day EVERY DAY!	
		_____ times per day EVERY DAY!	

Quick-Relief Medicines	How Much To Take	How Often	Other Instructions
		Take ONLY as needed	NOTE: If this medicine is needed frequently, call physician to consider increasing long-term-control medications.

Special instructions when I feel ● good, ○ not good, and ● awful.

GREEN ZONE — I feel good.
(My peak flow is in the GREEN zone.)

PREVENT asthma symptoms everyday:
☐ Take my long-term-control medicines (above) every day.
☐ Before exercise, take _____ puffs of _____
☐ Avoid things that make my asthma worse like: _____

YELLOW ZONE — I do *not* feel good.
(My peak flow is in the YELLOW zone.)
My symptoms may include one or more of the following:
- Wheeze
- Tight chest
- Cough
- Shortness of breath
- Waking up at night with asthma symptoms
- Decreased ability to do usual activities
- _____

CAUTION. I should continue taking my long-term-control asthma medicines every day AND:
☐ Take _____

If I still do not feel good, or my peak flow is not back in the *Green Zone* within 1 hour, then I should:
☐ Increase _____
☐ Add _____
☐ Call _____

RED ZONE — I feel *awful*.
(My peak flow is in the RED zone.)
Warning signs may include one or more of the following:
- It's getting harder and harder to breathe
- Unable to sleep or do usual activities because of trouble breathing

MEDICAL ALERT! Get help!
☐ Take _____ until I get help immediately.
☐ Take _____
☐ Call _____

Danger! Get help immediately! Call 9-1-1 if you have trouble walking or talking due to shortness of breath or lips or fingernails are gray or blue.

Adapted and reprinted with permission from the Regional Asthma Management and Prevention (RAMP) Initiative, a program of the Public Health Institute, to include terms used in the EPR—3: Full Report 2007.

Source: http://www.calasthma.org/uploads/resources/actionplanpdf.pdf; San Francisco Bay Area Regional Asthma Management Plan, http://www.rampasthma.org

FIGURE 6. SAMPLE ASTHMA ACTION PLAN—CHILD

ENGLISH

Child Asthma Action Plan
0–5 years of age

Patient Name: _____

Medical Record #: _____

Health Care Provider's Name: _____   DOB: _____

Health Care Provider's Phone #: _____   Completed by: _____   Date: _____

Long-Term-Control Medicines (Use Every Day To Stay Healthy)	How Much To Take	How Often	Other Instructions (such as spacers/masks, nebulizers)
		_____ times per day EVERY DAY!	
		_____ times per day EVERY DAY!	
		_____ times per day EVERY DAY!	
		_____ times per day EVERY DAY!	

Quick-Relief Medicines	How Much To Take	How Often	Other Instructions
		Give ONLY as needed	NOTE: If this medicine is needed often (_____ times per week), call physician.

GREEN ZONE

*Child is **well*** and has no asthma symptoms, even during active play.

PREVENT asthma symptoms every day:
- Give the above long-term-control medicines every day.
- Avoid things that make the child's asthma worse:
☑ Avoid tobacco smoke; ask people to smoke outside.
☐ _____
☐ _____

YELLOW ZONE

*Child is **not well*** and has asthma symptoms that may include:
- Coughing
- Wheezing
- Runny nose or other cold symptoms
- Breathing harder or faster
- Awakening due to coughing or difficulty breathing
- Playing less than usual
- _____
- _____

Other symptoms that could indicate that your child is having trouble breathing may include: difficulty feeding (grunting sounds, poor sucking), changes in sleep patterns, cranky and tired, decreased appetite.

CAUTION. Take action by continuing to give regular asthma medicines every day AND:

☐ Give _____
(include dose and frequency)

If the child is not in the *Green Zone* and still has symptoms after 1 hour, then:

☐ Give more _____
(include dose and frequency)

☐ _____
(include dose and frequency)

☐ Call _____

RED ZONE

*Child **feels awful!*** Warning signs may include:
- Child's wheeze, cough, or difficulty breathing continues or worsens, even after giving yellow zone medicines.
- Child's breathing is so hard that he/she is having trouble walking/talking/eating/playing.
- Child is drowsy or less alert than normal.

Danger! Get help immediately!

MEDICAL ALERT! Get help!
☐ Take the child to the hospital or call 9-1-1 immediately!
☐ Give more _____ until you get help. (include dose and frequency)
☐ Give _____ (include dose and frequency)

Call 9-1-1 if:
- The child's skin is sucked in around neck and ribs, or
- Lips and/or fingernails are grey or blue, or
- Child doesn't respond to you.

Adapted and reprinted with permission from "The Asthma Action Plan" developed by a committee facilitated by the Regional Asthma Management and Prevention (RAMP) Initiative, a program of the Public Health Institute.

Source: http://www.calasthma.org/uploads/resources/actionplanpdf.pdf; San Francisco Bay Area Regional Asthma Management Plan, http://www.rampasthma.org

FIGURE 7. DELIVERY OF ASTHMA EDUCATION BY CLINICIANS DURING PATIENT CARE VISITS

Assessment Questions	Information	Skills
Recommendations for Initial Visit		
Focus on: ■ Expectations of visit ■ Asthma control ■ Patients' goals of treatment ■ Medications ■ Quality of life **Ask relevant questions** "What worries you most about your asthma?" "What do you want to accomplish at this visit?" "What do you want to be able to do that you can't do now because of your asthma?" "What do you expect from treatment?" "What medicines have you tried?" "What other questions do you have for me today?" "Are there things in your environment that make your asthma worse?"	**Teach in simple language:** ■ What is asthma? Asthma is a chronic lung disease. The airways are very sensitive. They become inflamed and narrow; breathing becomes difficult. ■ The definition of asthma control: few daytime symptoms, no nighttime awakenings due to asthma, able to engage in normal activities, normal lung function. ■ Asthma treatments: two types of medicines are needed: — Long-term control: medications that prevent symptoms, often by reducing inflammation. — Quick relief: short-acting bronchodilator relaxes muscles around airways. ■ Bring all medications to every appointment. ■ When to seek medical advice. Provide appropriate telephone number.	**Teach or review and demonstrate:** ■ Inhaler and spacer or valved holding chamber (VHC) use. Check performance. ■ Self-monitoring skills that are tied to a written asthma action plan: — Recognize intensity and frequency of asthma symptoms. — Review the signs of deterioration and the need to reevaluate therapy: • Waking at night or early morning with asthma • Increased medication use • Decreased activity tolerance ■ Use of a written asthma action plan (See figures 5 and 6.) that includes instructions for daily management and for recognizing and handling worsening asthma.
Recommendations for First Followup Visit (2 to 4 Weeks or Sooner as Needed)		
Focus on: ■ Expectations of visit ■ Asthma control ■ Patient's goals of treatment ■ Medications ■ Patient's treatment preferences ■ Quality of life **Ask relevant questions from previous visit and also ask:** "What medications are you taking?" "How and when are you taking them?" "What problems have you had using your medications?" "Please show me how you use your inhaled medications."	**Teach in simple language:** ■ Use of two types of medications. ■ Remind patient to bring all medications and the peak flow meter, if using, to every appointment for review. ■ Self/assessment of asthma control using symptoms and/or peak flow as a guide.	**Teach or review and demonstrate:** ■ Use of written asthma action plan. Review and adjust as needed. ■ Peak flow monitoring if indicated ■ Correct inhaler and spacer or VHC technique.
Recommendations for Second Followup Visit		
Focus on: ■ Expectations of visit ■ Asthma control ■ Patients' goals of treatment ■ Medications ■ Quality of life **Ask relevant questions from previous visits and also ask:** "Have you noticed anything in your home, work, or school that makes your asthma worse?" "Describe for me how you know when to call your doctor or go to the hospital for asthma care." "What questions do you have about the asthma action plan?" "Can we make it easier?" "Are your medications causing you any problems?" "Have you noticed anything in your environment that makes your asthma worse?" "Have you missed any of your medications?"	**Teach in simple language:** ■ Self-assessment of asthma control, using symptoms and/or peak flow as a guide. ■ Relevant environmental control/avoidance strategies: — How to identify home, work, or school exposures that can cause or worsen asthma — How to control house-dust mites, animal exposures if applicable — How to avoid cigarette smoke (active and passive) ■ Review all medications.	**Teach or review and demonstrate:** ■ Inhaler/spacer or VHC technique. ■ Peak flow monitoring technique. ■ Use of written asthma action plan. Review and adjust as needed. ■ Confirm that patient knows what to do if asthma gets worse

FIGURE 7. DELIVERY OF ASTHMA EDUCATION BY CLINICIANS DURING PATIENT CARE VISITS (continued)

Assessment Questions	Information	Skills
Recommendations for All Subsequent Visits		
Focus on: - Expectations of visit - Asthma control - Patients' goals of treatment - Medications - Quality of life **Ask relevant questions from previous visits and also ask:** "How have you tried to control things that make your asthma worse?" "Please show me how you use your inhaled medication."	**Teach in simple language:** - Review and reinforce all: — Educational messages — Environmental control strategies at home, work, or school — Medications — Self-assessment of asthma control, using symptoms and/or peak flow as a guide	**Teach or review and demonstrate:** - Inhaler/spacer or VHC technique. - Peak flow monitoring technique, if appropriate. - Use of written asthma action plan. Review and adjust as needed. - Confirm that patient knows what to do if asthma gets worse.

Sources: Adapted from Guevara et al. 2003; Janson et al. 2003; Powell and Gibson 2003; Wilson et al. 1993.

---

such as interactive formats, practice-based case studies, and multidimensional teaching approaches that reinforce guideline-based care.

- Providing communication skills training to clinicians to enhance competence in caring for all patients, especially multicultural populations.

- Using systems approaches, such as clinical pathways and clinical information system prompts, to improve the quality of asthma care and to support clinical care decisionmaking.

Component 3: Control of Environmental Factors and Comorbid Conditions That Affect Asthma

If patients who have asthma are exposed to irritants or inhalant allergens to which they are sensitive, their asthma symptoms may increase and precipitate an asthma exacerbation. Substantially reducing exposure to these factors may reduce inflammation, symptoms, and need for medication. Several comorbid conditions can impede asthma management. Recognition and treatment of these conditions may improve asthma control. See questions in figure 3, "Suggested Items for Medical History," above, for questions related to environmental exposures and comorbid conditions.

Allergens and Irritants

Evaluate the potential role of allergens (particularly inhalant allergens) and irritants.

- Identify allergen and pollutants or irritant exposures. The most important allergens for both children and adults appear to be those that are inhaled.

- For patients who have persistent asthma, use skin testing or in vitro testing to assess sensitivity to perennial indoor allergens. Assess the significance of positive tests in the context of the person's history of symptoms when exposed to the allergen.

Advise patients who have asthma to reduce exposure to allergens and pollutants or irritants to which they are sensitive.

- See figure 9, "How To Control Things That Make Your Asthma Worse," for a sample patient information sheet.

- Effective allergen avoidance requires a multifaceted, comprehensive approach; single steps alone are generally ineffective. Multifaceted allergen-control education programs provided in the home setting can help patients reduce exposures to cockroach, dust-mite, and rodent allergens and, consequently, improve asthma control.

- Advise patients who have severe persistent asthma, nasal polyps, or a history of sensitivity to aspirin or nonsteroidal anti-inflammatory drugs (NSAIDs) about their risk of severe and even fatal exacerbations from using these drugs.

- Indoor air-cleaning devices (high-efficiency particulate air [HEPA] and electrostatic precipitating filters), cannot substitute for more effective dust-mite and cockroach control measures because

FIGURE 8. ASTHMA EDUCATION RESOURCES

Allergy & Asthma Network Mothers of Asthmatics 1-800-878-4403
2751 Prosperity Avenue, Suite 150 1-703-641-9595
Fairfax, VA 22030
www.breatherville.org

American Academy of Allergy, Asthma and Immunology 1-414-272-6071
555 East Wells Street, Suite 100
Milwaukee, WI 53202-3823
www.aaaai.org

American Association For Respiratory Care 1-972-243-2272
9125 North MacArthur Boulevard, Suite 100
Irving, TX 75063
www.aarc.org

American College of Allergy, Asthma, and Immunology 1-800-842-7777
85 West Algonquin Road 1-847-427-1200
Suite 550
Arlington Heights, IL 60005
www.Acaai.Org

American Lung Association 1-800-586-4872
61 Broadway
New York, NY 10006
www.lungusa.org

Association of Asthma Educators 1-888-988-7747
1215 Anthony Avenue
Columbia, SC 29201
www.asthmaeducators.org

Asthma and Allergy Foundation of America 1-800-727-8462
1233 20th Street, NW., Suite 402
Washington, DC 20036
www.aafa.org

Centers for Disease Control and Prevention 1-800-311-3435
1600 Clifton Road
Atlanta, GA 30333

Food Allergy & Anaphylaxis Network 1-800-929-4040
11781 Lee Jackson Highway, Suite 160
Fairfax, VA 22033
www.foodallergy.org

National Heart, Lung, and Blood Institute Information Center 1-301-592-8573
P.O. Box 30105
Bethesda, MD 20824-0105
www.nhlbi.nih.gov

National Jewish Medical and Research Center (Lung Line) 1-800-222-Lung
1400 Jackson Street
Denver, CO 80206
www.njc.org

U.S. Environmental Protection Agency 1-800-490-9198
National Center for Environmental Publications
P.O. Box 42419
Cincinnati, OH 45242-0419
www.airnow.gov

these particles do not remain airborne. The devices can reduce airborne dog and cat allergens, mold spores, and particulate tobacco smoke; however, most studies do not show an effect on symptoms or lung function.

- Use of humidifiers or evaporative (swamp) coolers is not generally recommended in homes of patients who are sensitive to dust mites or mold.

Consider subcutaneous allergen immunotherapy for patients who have persistent asthma when there is clear evidence of a relationship between symptoms and exposure to an allergen to which the patient is sensitive. Evidence is strongest for use of subcutaneous immunotherapy for single allergens, particularly house dust mites, animal dander, and pollen. The role of allergy in asthma is greater in children than in adults. If use of allergen immunotherapy is elected, it should be administered only in a physician's office where facilities and trained personnel are available to treat any life-threatening reaction that can, but rarely does, occur.

Consider inactivated influenza vaccination for patients who have asthma. This vaccine is safe for administration to children over 6 months of age and adults, and the Advisory Committee on Immunization Practices of the Centers for Disease Control and Prevention (CDC) recommends vaccination for persons who have asthma because they are considered to be at risk for complications from influenza. However, the vaccine should not be given with the expectation that it will reduce either the frequency or severity of asthma exacerbations during the influenza season.

Dietary factors have an inconclusive role in asthma. Food allergenies are rarely an aggravating factor in asthma. An exception is that sulfites in foods (e.g., shrimp, dried fruit, processed potatoes, beer, and wine) can precipitate asthma symptoms in people who are sensitive to these food items. Furthermore, individuals who have both food allergy and asthma are at increased risk for fatal anaphlylactic reactions to the food to which they are sensitized.

Comorbid Conditions

Identify and treat comorbid conditions that may impede asthma management. If these conditions are treated appropriately, asthma control may improve.

- **Allergic Bronchopulmonary Aspergillosis (ABPA)** may be considered in patients who have asthma and a history of pulmonary infiltrates, immunoglobulin E (IgE) sensitization to Aspergillus, and/or are corticosteroid dependent. Diagnostic criteria include: positive immediate skin test and elevated serum IgE and/or IgG to Aspergillus, total serum IgE >417 IU (1,000 ng/mL), and central bronchiectasis. Treatment is prednisone, initially 0.5 mg per kilogram with gradual tapering. Azole antifungal agents as adjunctive therapy may also be helpful.

- **Gastroesophageal Reflux (GERD)** treatment may benefit patients who have asthma and complain of frequent heartburn or pyrosis, particularly those who have frequent nighttime asthma symptoms. Even in the absence of suggestive GERD symptoms, consider evaluation for GERD in patients who have poorly controlled asthma, especially with nighttime symptoms. Treatment includes: avoiding heavy meals, fried foods, caffeine, and alcohol; avoiding food and drink within 3 hours of retiring; elevating the head of the bed on 6- to 8-inch blocks; using proton pump inhibitor medication.

- **Obese or overweight patients** who have asthma may be advised that weight loss, in addition to improving overall health, might also improve asthma control.

- **Obstructive Sleep Apnea (OSA)** may be considered in patients who have not well controlled asthma, particularly those who are overweight or obese. Treatment for OSA is nasal continuous positive air way pressure (CPAP). However, this treatment may disrupt the sleep of asthma patients who do not also have OSA. Accurate diagnosis is important.

- **Rhinitis or sinusitis** symptoms or diagnosis should be evaluated in patients who have asthma, because the interrelationship of the upper and lower airway suggests that therapy for the upper airway will improve asthma control. Treatment of allergic rhinitis includes intranasal corticosteroids, antihistamine therapy, and the consideration of immunotherapy. Treatment of sinusitis includes intranasal corticosteroids and antibiotics. Evidence is inconclusive regarding the effect on asthma of sinus surgery in patients who have chronic rhinosinusitis.

- **Stress and depression** should be considered in patients who have asthma that is not well controlled. Additional education to improve self-management and coping skills may be helpful.

FIGURE 9. HOW TO CONTROL THINGS THAT MAKE YOUR ASTHMA WORSE

You can help prevent asthma episodes by staying away from things that make your asthma worse. This guide suggests many ways to help you do this.

You need to find out what makes your asthma worse. Some things that make asthma worse for some people are not a problem for others. You do not need to do all of the things listed in this guide.

Look at the things listed below. Put a check next to the ones that you know make your asthma worse, particularly if you are allergic to these things. Then, decide with your doctor what steps you will take. Start with the things in your bedroom that bother your asthma. Try something simple first.

Tobacco Smoke

- ☐ If you smoke, ask your doctor for ways to help you quit. Ask family members to quit smoking, too.
- ☐ Do not allow smoking in your home, car or around you.
- ☐ Be sure no one smokes at a child's daycare center or school.

Dust Mites

Many people who have asthma are allergic to dust mites. Dust mites are like tiny "bugs" you cannot see that live in cloth or carpet.

Things that will help the most:
- ☐ Encase your mattress in a special dust-mite proof cover.*
- ☐ Encase your pillow in a special dust-mite proof cover* or wash the pillow each week in hot water. Water must be hotter than 130 °F to kill the mites. Cooler water used with detergent and bleach can also be effective.
- ☐ Wash the sheets and blankets on your bed each week in hot water.

Other things that can help:
- ☐ Reduce indoor humidity to or below 60 percent, ideally 30–50 percent. Dehumidifiers or central air conditioners can do this.
- ☐ Try not to sleep or lie on cloth-covered cushions or furniture.
- ☐ Remove carpets from your bedroom and those laid on concrete, if you can.
- ☐ Keep stuffed toys out of the bed, or wash the toys weekly in hot water or in cooler water with detergent and bleach. Placing toys weekly in a dryer or freezer may help. Prolonged exposure to dry heat or freezing can kill mites but does not remove allergen.

*To find out where to get products mentioned in this guide, call:

Asthma and Allergy Foundation of America (800–727–8462)

Allergy & Asthma Network Mothers of Asthmatics (800–878–4403)

American Academy of Allergy, Asthma, and Immunology (800–822–2762)

National Jewish Medical and Research Center (Lung Line) (800–222–5864)

American College of Allergy, Asthma, and Immunology (800–842–7777)

Animal Dander

Some people are allergic to the flakes of skin or dried saliva from animals.

The best thing to do:
- Keep pets with fur or hair out of your home.

If you can't keep the pet outdoors, then:
- Keep the pet out of your bedroom, and keep the bedroom door closed.
- Remove carpets and furniture covered with cloth from your home. If that is not possible, keep the pet out of the rooms where these are.

Cockroach

Many people with asthma are allergic to the dried droppings and remains of cockroaches.

- Keep all food out of your bedroom.
- Keep food and garbage in closed containers (Never leave food out).
- Use poison baits, powders, gels, or paste (for example, boric acid). You can also use traps.
- If a spray is used to kill roaches, stay out of the room until the odor goes away.

Vacuum Cleaning

- Try to get someone else to vacuum for you once or twice a week, if you can. Stay out of rooms while they are being vacuumed and for a short while afterward.
- If you vacuum, use a dust mask (from a hardware store), a central cleaner with the collecting bag outside the home, or a vacuum cleaner with a HEPA filter or a double-layered bag.*

Indoor Mold

- Fix leaking faucets, pipes, or other sources of water.
- Clean moldy surfaces.
- Dehumidify basements if possible.

Pollen and Outdoor Mold

During your allergy season (when pollen or mold spore counts are high):
- Try to keep your windows closed.
- If possible, stay indoors with windows closed during the midday and afternoon, if you can. Pollen and some mold spore counts are highest at that time.
- Ask your doctor whether you need to take or increase anti-inflammatory medicine before your allergy season starts.

Smoke, Strong Odors, and Sprays

- If possible, do not use a wood-burning stove, kerosene heater, fireplace, unvented gas stove, or heater.
- Try to stay away from strong odors and sprays, such as perfume, talcum powder, hair spray, paints, new carpet, or particle board.

Exercise or Sports

- You should be able to be active without symptoms. See your doctor if you have asthma symptoms when you are active—such as when you exercise, do sports, play, or work hard.
- Ask your doctor about taking medicine before you exercise to prevent symptoms.
- Warm up for a period before you exercise.
- Check the air quality index and try not to work or play hard outside when the air pollution or pollen levels (if you are allergic to the pollen) are high.

Other Things That Can Make Asthma Worse

- **Sulfites in foods:** Do not drink beer or wine or eat shrimp, dried fruit, or processed potatoes if they cause asthma symptoms.
- **Cold air:** Cover your nose and mouth with a scarf on cold or windy days.
- **Other medicines:** Tell your doctor about all the medicines you may take. Include cold medicines, aspirin, and even eye drops.

Key: HEPA, high-efficiency particulate air

Component 4: Medications

Medications for asthma are categorized into two general classes: long-term control medication and quick-relief medication. Selection of medications includes consideration of the general mechanisms and role of the medication in therapy, delivery devices, and safety.

General Mechanisms and Role in Therapy

Long-term control medications are used daily to achieve and maintain control of persistent asthma. The most effective are those that attenuate the underlying inflammation characteristic of asthma. Long-term control medications include the following (listed in alphabetical order):

- **Corticosteroids** are anti-inflammatory medications that reduce airway hyperresponsiveness, inhibit inflammatory cell migration and activation, and block late phase reaction to allergen. Inhaled Corticosteriods (ICSs) are the most consistently effective long-term control medication at all steps of care for persistent asthma, and ICSs improve asthma control more effectively in both children and adults than leukotriene receptor antagonists (LTRAs) or any other single, long-term control medication do. ICSs reduce impairment and risk of exacerbations, but ICSs do not appear to alter the progression or underlying severity of the disease in children. Short courses of oral systemic corticosteroids are often used to gain prompt control of asthma. Oral systemic corticosteroids are used long term to treat patients who require step 6 care (for severe persistent asthma).

- **Cromolyn sodium and nedocromil** stabilize mast cells and interfere with chloride channel function. They are used as alternative, but not preferred, medication for patients requiring step 2 care (for mild persistent asthma). They also can be used as preventive treatment before exercise or unavoidable exposure to known allergens.

- **Immunomodulators.** Omalizumab (anti-IgE) is a monoclonal antibody that prevents binding of IgE to the high-affinity receptors on basophils and mast cells. Omalizumab is used as adjunctive therapy for patients 12 years of age who have sensitivity to relevant allergens (e.g., dust mite, cockroach, cat, or dog) and who require step 5 or 6 care (for severe persistent asthma). Clinicians who administer omalizumab should be prepared and equipped to identify and treat anaphylaxis that may occur.

- **Leukotriene modifiers** interfere with the pathway of leukotriene mediators, which are released from mast cells, eosinophils, and basophils. These medications include LTRAs (montelukast and zafirlukast) and a 5-lipoxygenase inhibitor (zileuton). LTRAs are alternative, but not preferred, therapy for the treatment of patients who require step 2 care (for mild persistent asthma). LTRAs also can be used as adjunctive therapy with ICSs, but for youths 12 years of age and adults, they are not preferred adjunctive therapy compared to the addition of LABAs. LTRAs can attenuate EIB. Zileuton can be used as alternative, but not preferred, adjunctive therapy in adults; liver function monitoring is essential.

- **LABAs** (salmeterol and formoterol) are inhaled bronchodilators that have a duration of bronchodilation of at least 12 hours after a single dose.

    — LABAs are not to be used as monotherapy for long-term control of asthma.

    — LABAs are used in combination with ICSs for long-term control and prevention of symptoms in moderate or severe persistent asthma (Step 3 care or higher in children ≥5 years of age and adults and Step 4 care or higher in children 0–4 years of age, although few data are available for 0–4-year-olds.).

    — Of the adjunctive therapies available, LABA is the preferred therapy to combine with ICS in youths ≥12 years of age and adults.

    — A LABA may be used before exercise to prevent EIB, but duration of action does not exceed 5 hours with chronic, regular use. Frequent or chronic use before exercise is discouraged, because this may disguise poorly controlled persistent asthma. See also the section "Safety Issues for Inhaled Corticosteroids and Long-Acting Beta$_2$-Agonists."

- **Methylxanthines.** Sustained-release theophylline is a mild to moderate bronchodilator used as alternative, not preferred, therapy for step 2 care (for mild persistent asthma) or as adjunctive therapy with ICS in patients ≥5 years of age. Theophylline may have mild anti-inflammatory effects. Monitoring of serum theophylline concentration is essential.

Quick-relief medications are used to treat acute symptoms and exacerbations. They include the following (listed in alphabetical order):

- **Anticholinergics** inhibit muscarinic cholinergic receptors and reduce intrinsic vagal tone of the airway. Ipratropium bromide provides additive benefit to SABA in moderate or severe exacerbations in the emergency care setting, not the hospital setting. Ipratropium bromide may be used as an alternative bronchodilator for patients who do not tolerate SABA, although it has not been compared to SABAs.

- **SABAs**—albuterol, levalbuterol, and pirbuterol—are bronchodilators that relax smooth muscle. They are the treatment of choice for relief of acute symptoms and prevention of EIB. Increasing use of SABA treatment or the use of SABA >2 days a week for symptom relief (not prevention of EIB) generally indicates inadequate asthma control and the need for initiating or intensifying anti-inflammatory therapy. Regularly scheduled, daily, chronic use of SABA is not recommended.

- **Systemic corticosteroids.** Although not short-acting, oral systemic corticosteroids are used for moderate and severe exacerbations in addition to SABA to speed recovery and to prevent recurrence of exacerbations.

Complementary and alternative medications (CAMs) and interventions generally have insufficient evidence to permit recommendations. Because as much as one-third of the U.S. population uses complementary alternative healing methods, it is important to discuss their use with patients.

- **Ask patients about all the medications and interventions they are using.** Some cultural beliefs and practices may be of no harm and can be integrated into the recommended asthma management strategies, but it is important to advise patients that alternative healing methods are not substitutes for recommended therapeutic approaches. Clinical trials on safety and efficacy are limited, and their scientific basis has not been established.

- **Evidence is insufficient to recommend or not recommend most CAMs or treatments for asthma.** These include chiropractic therapy, homeopathy and herbal medicine, and breathing or relaxation techniques. Acupuncture is not recommended for the treatment of asthma.

- **Patients who use herbal treatments for asthma should be cautioned** about the potential for harmful ingredients and for interactions with recommended asthma medications.

Delivery Devices for Inhaled Medications

Patients should be instructed in the use of inhaled medications, and patients' technique should be reviewed at every patient visit. The major advantages of delivering drugs directly into the lungs via inhalation are that higher concentrations can be delivered more effectively to the airways and that systemic side effects are lessened. Inhaled medications, or aerosols, are available in a variety of devices that differ in the technique required. See figure 10, "Aerosol Delivery Devices," for a summary of issues to consider for different devices.

Safety Issues for Inhaled Corticosteroids and Long-Acting Beta$_2$-Agonists

Inhaled Corticosteroids

- ICSs are the preferred long-term control therapy in children of all ages and adults. In general, ICSs are well tolerated and safe at the recommended dosages.

- Most benefits of ICS for patients who have mild or moderate asthma occur at the low- to medium-dose ranges. Data suggest higher doses may further reduce the risk of exacerbations. Furthermore, higher doses are beneficial for patients who have more severe asthma. The risk of adverse effects increases with the dose.

- High doses of ICS administered for prolonged periods of time (e.g., >1 year) have significantly less potential than oral systemic corticosteroids for having adverse effects. High doses of ICS used for prolonged periods of time (e.g., >1 year), particularly in combination with frequent courses of oral corticosteroids, may be associated with risk of posterior subcapsular cataracts or reduced bone density. Slit-lamp eye exam and bone densitometry may be considered. For adult patients, consider supplements of calcium and vitamin D, particularly in perimenopausal women. For children, age-appropriate dietary intake of calcium and vitamin D should be reviewed with parents or caregivers.

- To reduce the potential for adverse effects, the following measures are recommended.

    — Advise patients to use spacers or VHCs with nonbreath-activated metered-dose inhalers

(MDIs) to reduce local side effects. There are no clinical data on use of spacers with ultrafine particle hydrofluoroalkane (HFA) MDIs.

— Advise patients to rinse the mouth (rinse and spit) after inhalation.

— Use the lowest dose of ICS that maintains asthma control. Evaluate the patient's inhaler technique and adherence, as well as environmental control measures, before increasing the dose.

— Consider adding a LABA, or alternative adjunctive therapy, to a low or medium dose of ICS rather than using a higher dose of ICS to maintain asthma control.

Inhaled Corticosteroids and Linear Growth in Children

- The potential risks of ICSs are well balanced by their benefits.

- Poorly controlled asthma may delay growth. Children who have asthma tend to have longer periods of reduced growth rates before puberty.

- Growth rates are highly variable in children. Short-term evaluation may not be predictive of final adult height attained.

- The potential for adverse effects on linear growth from ICS appear to be dose dependent. In treatment of children who have mild or moderate persistent asthma, low-to medium-dose ICS therapy may be associated with a possible, but not predictable, adverse effect on linear growth (approximately 1 cm). The effect on growth velocity appears to occur in the first several months of treatment and is generally small and not progressive. The clinical significance of this potential systemic effect has yet to be determined.

- In general, the efficacy of ICSs is sufficient to outweigh any concerns about growth or other systemic effects. However, ICSs should be titrated to as low a dose as needed to maintain good control of the child's asthma, and children receiving ICSs should be monitored for changes in growth by using a stadiometer.

Long-Acting Beta2-Agonists

- The addition of LABA (salmeterol or formoterol) to the treatment of patients who require more than low-dose ICS alone to control asthma improves lung function, decreases symptoms, reduces exacerbations and use of SABA for quick relief in most patients to a greater extent than doubling the dose of ICSs.

- A large clinical trial comparing daily treatment with salmeterol or placebo added to usual asthma therapy resulted in an increased risk of asthma-related deaths in patients treated with salmeterol (13 deaths among 13,176 patients treated for 28 weeks with salmeterol versus 3 deaths among 13,179 patients treated with placebo). In addition, increased numbers of severe asthma exacerbations were noted in the pivotal trials submitted to the U.S. Food and Drug Administration (FDA) for formoterol approval, particularly in the arms of the trials with higher dose formoterol. Thus, the FDA determined that a Black Box warning was warranted on all preparations containing a LABA.

- The established beneficial effects of LABA for the great majority of patients who require more therapy than low-dose ICS alone to control asthma (i.e., require step 3 care or higher) should be weighed against the increased risk for severe exacerbations, although uncommon, associated with the daily use of LABAs.

- Daily use of LABA generally should not exceed 100 mcg salmeterol or 24 mcg formoterol.

- It is not currently recommended that LABA be used for treatment of acute symptoms or exacerbations.

- LABAs are not to be used as monotherapy for long-term control. Patients should be instructed not to stop ICS therapy while taking LABA, even though their symptoms may significantly improve.

Stepwise Approach for Managing Asthma

Principles of The Stepwise Approach

A stepwise approach to managing asthma is recommended to gain and maintain control of asthma in both the impairment and risk domains. These domains may respond differentially to treatment.

For children, see:

Figure 11, "Classifying Asthma Severity and Initiating Therapy in Children"

FIGURE 10. AEROSOL DELIVERY DEVICES

Device/Drugs	Population	Optimal Technique*	Therapeutic Issues
Metered-dose inhaler (MDI) Beta$_2$-agonists Corticosteroids Cromolyn sodium Anticholinergics	≥5 years old (<5 with spacer or valved holding chamber (VHC) or mask)	Actuation during a slow (30 L/min or 3–5 seconds) deep inhalation, followed by 10-second breathhold. Under laboratory conditions, open-mouth technique (holding MDI 2 inches away from open mouth) enhances delivery to the lung. This technique, however, has not been shown to enhance clinical benefit consistently compared to closed-mouth technique (inserting MDI mouthpiece between lips and teeth).	Slow inhalation and coordination of actuation during inhalation may be difficult, particularly in young children and elderly. Patients may incorrectly stop inhalation at actuation. Deposition of 50–80 percent of actuated dose in oropharynx. Mouth washing and spitting is effective in reducing the amount of drug swallowed and absorbed systemically. Lung delivery under ideal conditions varies significantly between MDIs due to differences in formulation (suspension versus solution), propellant (chlorofluorocarbon [CFC] versus hydrofluoralkane [HFA]), and valve design. For example, inhaled corticosteroid (ICS) delivery varies from 5–50 percent.
Breath-actuated MDI Beta$_2$-agonist	≥5 years old	Tight seal around mouthpiece and slightly more rapid inhalation than standard MDI (see above) followed by 10-second breathhold.	May be particularly useful for patients unable to coordinate inhalation and actuation. May also be useful for elderly patients. Patients may incorrectly stop inhalation at actuation. Cannot be used with currently available spacer/valved holding chamber (VHC) devices.
Dry powder inhaler (DPI) Beta$_2$-agonists Corticosteroids Anticholinergics	≥4 years old	Rapid (60 L/min or 1–2 seconds), deep inhalation. Minimally effective inspiratory flow is device dependent. Most children <4 years of age may not generate sufficient inspiratory flow to activate the inhaler.	Dose is lost if patient exhales through device after actuating. Delivery may be greater or lesser than MDI, depending on device and technique. Delivery is more flow dependent in devices with highest internal resistance. Rapid inhalation promotes greater deposition in larger central airways. Mouth washing and spitting is effective in reducing amount of drug swallowed and absorbed.
Spacer or valved holding chamber (VHC)	≥4 years old <4 years old VHC with face mask	Slow (30 L/min or 3–5 seconds) deep inhalation, followed by 10-second breathhold immediately following actuation. Actuate only once into spacer/VHC per inhalation. If face mask is used, it should have a tight fit and allow 3–5 inhalations per actuation. Rinse plastic VHCs once a month with low concentration of liquid household dishwashing detergent (1:5,000 or 1–2 drops per cup of water) and let drip dry.	Indicated for patients who have difficulty performing adequate MDI technique. May be bulky. Simple tubes do not obviate coordinating actuation and inhalation. The VHCs are preferred. Face mask allows MDIs to be used with small children. However, use of a face mask reduces delivery to lungs by 50 percent. The VHC improves lung delivery and response in patients who have poor MDI technique. The effect of a spacer or VHC on output from an MDI depends on both the MDI and device type; thus data from one combination should not be extrapolated to all others. Spacers and/or VHCs decrease oropharyngeal deposition and thus decrease risk of topical side effects (e.g., thrush). Spacers will also reduce the potential systemic availability of ICSs with higher oral absorption. However, spacer/VHCs may increase systemic availability of ICSs that are poorly absorbed orally by enhancing delivery to lungs. No clinical data are available on use of spacers or VHCs with ultrafine-particle-generated HFA MDIs. Use anti-static VHCs or rinse plastic non-anti-static VHCs with dilute household detergents to enhance delivery to lungs and efficacy. This effect is less pronounced for albuterol MDIs with HFA propellant than for albuterol MDIs with CFC propellant. As effective as nebulizer for delivering SABAs and anticholinergics in mild- to moderate-exacerbations; data in severe exacerbations are limited.

FIGURE 10. AEROSOL DELIVERY DEVICES (continued)

Device/Drugs	Population	Optimal Technique*	Therapeutic Issues
Nebulizer Beta$_2$-agonists Corticosteroids Cromolyn sodium Anticholinergics	Patients of any age who cannot use MDI with VHC and face mask.	Slow tidal breathing with occasional deep breaths. Tightly fitting face mask for those unable to use mouthpiece. Using the "blow by" technique (i.e., holding the mask or open tube near the infant's nose and mouth) is not appropriate.	Less dependent on patient's coordination and cooperation. Delivery method of choice for cromolyn sodium in young children. May be expensive; time consuming; bulky; output is dependent on device and operating parameters (fill volume, driving gas flow); internebulizer and intranebulizer output variances are significant. Use of a face mask reduces delivery to lungs by 50 percent. Nebulizers are as effective as MDIs plus VHCs for delivering bronchodilators in the ED for mild to moderate exacerbations; data in severe exacerbations are limited. Choice of delivery system is dependent on resources, availability, and clinical judgment of the clinician caring for the patient. Potential for bacterial infections if not cleaned properly.

Key: ED, emergency department; SABAs, inhaled short-acting beta$_2$-agonists
*See figures in component 2—Education for a Partnership in Asthma Care for description of MDI and DPI techniques.

Figure 12, "Assessing Asthma Control and Adjusting Therapy in Children"

Figure 13, "Stepwise Approach for Managing Asthma Long Term in Children, 0–4 Years of Age and 5–11 Years of Age"

For adults, see:

Figure 14, "Classifying Asthma Severity and Initiating Treatment in Youths 12 Years of Age and Adults"

Figure 15, "Assessing Asthma Control and Adjusting Therapy in Youths ≥ 12 Years of Age and Adults"

Figure 16, "Stepwise Approach for Managing Asthma in Youths ≥12 Years of Age and Adults"

For medication dosages, see:

Figure 17, "Usual Dosages for Long-Term Control Medications"

Figure 18, "Estimated Comparative Daily Dosages for Inhaled Corticosteroids"

Figure 19, "Usual Dosages for Quick-Relief Medications"

- The stepwise approach incorporates all four components of care: assessment of severity to initiate therapy or assessment of control to monitor and adjust therapy; patient education; environmental control measures, and management of comorbid conditions at every step; and selection of medication.

- The type, amount, and scheduling of medication is determined by the level of asthma severity or asthma control.

  — Therapy is increased (stepped up) as necessary and decreased (stepped down) when possible.

  — Because asthma is a chronic inflammatory disorder, persistent asthma is most effectively controlled with daily long-term control medication directed toward suppressing inflammation. ICSs are the most consistently effective anti-inflammatory therapy for all age groups, at all steps of care for persistent asthma.

  — Selection among alternative treatment options is based on consideration of treatment effectiveness for the domain of particular relevance to the patient (impairment, risk, or both), the individual patient's history of previous response to therapies (sensitivity and responsiveness to different asthma medications can vary among patients), and the willingness and ability of the patient and family to use the medication.

- Once asthma control is achieved, monitoring and followup are essential, because asthma often varies over time. A step up in therapy may be needed, or a step down may be possible, to identify the minimum medication necessary to maintain control.

The stepwise approach and recommended treatments are meant to assist, not replace, the clinical decisionmaking necessary to determine the most appropriate treatment to meet the individual patient's needs and circumstances.

Referral to an asthma specialist for consultation or comanagement is recommended if there are difficulties achieving or maintaining control of asthma, if the patient required >2 bursts of oral systemic corticosteroids in 1 year or has an exacerbation requiring hospitalization, if step 4 care or higher is required (step 3 care or higher for children 0–4 years of age), if immunotherapy or omalizumab is considered, or if additional testing is indicated.

To achieve control of asthma, the following sequence of activities is recommended:

- For patients who are not already taking long-term control medications, assess asthma severity and initiate therapy according to the level of severity.

- For patients who are already taking long-term control medications, assess asthma control and step up therapy if the patient's asthma is not well controlled on current therapy. Before stepping up, review the patient's adherence to medications, inhaler technique, and environmental control measures.

- Evaluate asthma control in 2–6 weeks (depending on level of initial severity or control).

  — In general, classify the level of asthma control by the most severe indicator of impairment or risk.

  — The risk domain is usually more strongly associated with morbidity in young children than the impairment domain because young children are often symptom free between exacerbations.

  — If office spirometry suggests worse control than other measures of impairment, consider fixed obstruction and reassess the other measures. If fixed obstruction does not explain the lack of control, step up therapy, because low FEV_1 is a predictor of exacerbations.

  — If the history of exacerbations suggests poorer control than does assessment of impairment, reassess impairment measures, and consider a step up in therapy. Review plans for handling exacerbations and include the use of oral systemic corticosteroids, especially for patients who have a history of severe exacerbations.

- If asthma control is not achieved with the above actions:

  — Review the patient's adherence to medications, inhaler technique, environmental control measures (or whether there are new exposures), and management of comorbid conditions.

  — If adherence and environment control measures are adequate, then step up one step (if not well controlled) or two steps (if very poorly controlled).

  — If an alternative treatment was used initially, discontinue its use and use the preferred treatment option before stepping up therapy.

  — A short course of oral systemic corticosteroids may be considered to gain more rapid control for patients whose asthma frequently interrupts sleep or normal daily activities or who are experiencing an exacerbation at the time of assessment.

  — If lack of control persists, consider alternative diagnoses before stepping up further.

  — If the patient experiences side effects, consider different treatment options.

To maintain control of asthma, regular followup contact is essential because asthma often varies over time.

- Schedule patient contact at 1- to 6-month intervals; the interval will depend on such factors as the level or duration of asthma control and the level of treatment required.

- Consider a step down in therapy once asthma is well controlled for at least 3 months. A step down is necessary to identify the minimum therapy required to maintain good control. A reduction in therapy should be gradual and must be closely monitored. Studies are limited in guiding therapy reduction. In general, the dose of ICS may be reduced 25 percent to 50 percent every 3 months to the lowest possible dose.

- Consider seasonal periods of daily long-term control therapy for patients who have asthma symptoms only in relation to certain seasons (e.g., seasonal pollens, allergens, or viral respiratory infections) and who have intermittent asthma the rest of the year. This approach has not been rigorously evaluated; close monitoring for 2–6 weeks after therapy is discontinued is essential to assure sustained asthma control.

Stepwise Treatment Recommendations for Different Ages

Recommendations for treatments in the different steps are presented in three different age groups (0–4 years, 5–11 years, and 12 years and older) because the course of the disease may change over time, the relevance of measures of impairment or risk and the potential short- and long-term impact of medications may be age related, and varied levels of scientific evidence are available for the different ages.

Steps for Children 0–4 Years of Age

See figure 13, for recommended treatments in the different steps and figures 17–19 for recommended medication dosages. In addition to the general principles of the stepwise approach, special considerations for this age group include initiating therapy, selecting among treatment options, and monitoring response to therapy.

The initiation of daily long-term control therapy in children ages 0–4 years is recommended as follows:

- It is recommended for reducing impairment and risk of exacerbations in infants and young children who had four or more episodes of wheezing in the past year that lasted more than 1 day and affected sleep AND who have a positive asthma predictive index (either (1) one of the following: a parental history of asthma, a physician's diagnosis of atopic dermatitis, or evidence of sensitization to aeroallergens; OR (2) two of the following: evidence of sensitization to foods, >4 percent peripheral blood eosinophilia, or wheezing apart from colds).

- It should be considered for reducing impairment in infants and young children who consistently require symptomatic treatment >2 days per week for a period of more than 4 weeks.

- It should be considered for reducing risk in infants and young children who have two exacerbations requiring systemic corticosteroids within 6 months.

- It may be considered for use only during periods, or seasons, of previously documented risk (e.g., during seasons of viral respiratory infections).

The decision about when to start long-term daily therapy is difficult. The chronic airway inflammatory response in asthma can develop in the preschool years; for example, between 50–80 percent of children who have asthma developed symptoms before their fifth birthday. Adequate treatment will reduce the burden of illness, and underdiagnosis and undertreatment are key problems in this age group. Not all wheeze and cough are caused by asthma, however, and caution is needed to avoid giving inappropriate, prolonged therapy.

Initiating long-term control therapy will depend on consideration of issues regarding diagnosis and prognosis.

— Viral respiratory infections are the most common cause of asthma symptoms in this age group, and many children who wheeze with respiratory infections respond well to asthma therapy even though the diagnosis of asthma is not clearly established. For children who have exacerbations with viral infections, exacerbations are often severe (requiring emergency care or hospitalization), yet the child has no significant symptoms in between these exacerbations. These children have a low level of impairment but a high level of risk.

— Most young children who wheeze with viral respiratory infection experience a remission of symptoms by 6 years of age, perhaps due to growing airway size.

— However, two-thirds of children who have frequent wheezing AND also have a positive asthma predictive index (see above) are likely to have asthma throughout childhood. Early identification of these children allows appropriate treatment with environmental control measures and medication to reduce morbidity.

Select medications with the following considerations for young children:

- Asthma treatment for young children, especially infants, has not been studied adequately. Most recommendations are based on limited data and extrapolations from studies in older children and adults. Preferred treatment options are based on individual drug efficacy studies in this age group; comparator trials are not available.

- The following long-term control medications are FDA approved for the following ages in young children: ICS budesonide nebulizer solution (1–8 years of age); ICS fluticasone dry power inhaler (DPI) (>4 years of age); LABA salmeterol DPI, alone or in combination with ICS (>4 years of age); LTRA montelukast (chewable tablets, 2–6 years of age; granules, down to 1 year old).

- Several delivery devices are available, and the doses received may vary considerably among devices and age groups. In general, children <4 years of age will have less difficulty with a face mask and either (1) a nebulizer or (2) an MDI with a VHC. (See figure 10 above.)

- ICSs are the preferred long-term control medication for initiating therapy. The benefits of ICSs out weigh any concerns about potential risks of a small, nonprogressive reduction in growth velocity or other possible adverse effects. ICSs, as with all medications, should be titrated to as low a dose as needed to maintain control.

- For children whose asthma is not well controlled on low-dose ICS, few studies are available on stepup therapy in this age group, and the studies have mixed findings. Some data on children ≤4 years old and younger show dose-dependent improvements in the domains of impairment and risk of exacerbation from taking ICS. Data from studies on LABA combined with ICS have only small numbers of 4-year-old children, and these data show improvement in the impairment but not risk domain. Adding a noncorticosteroid long-term control medication to medium-dose ICS may be considered before increasing the dose of ICS to high dose to avoid potential risk of side effects with high doses of medication.

Monitor response to therapy closely, because treatment of young children is often in the form of a therapeutic trial.

- **If a clear and beneficial response is not obvious within 4–6 weeks and the patient's/family's medication technique and adherence are satisfactory, treatment should be stopped. Alternative therapies or alternative diagnoses should be considered.**

- **If a clear and beneficial response is sustained for at least 3 months, consider a step down to evaluate the need for continued daily long-term control therapy.** Children in this age group have high rates of spontaneous remission of symptoms.

Steps for Children 5–11 Years of Age

See figure 13, "Stepwise Approach for Managing Asthma Long Term in Children, 0–4 Years of Age and 5–11 Years of Age," for recommended treatments in different steps and figures 17, 18, and 19 for recommended medication dosages. Special considerations for this age group include the following:

Promote active participation in physical activities, exercise, and sports because physical activity is an essential part of a child's life. Treatment immediately before vigorous activity usually prevents EIB (see section on "Exercise-Induced Bronchospasm"). However, if the child has poor endurance or has symptoms during usual play activities, a step up in therapy is warranted.

Directly involve children ≥10 years of age (and younger children as appropriate) in developing their written asthma action plans and reviewing their adherence. This involvement may help address developmental issues of emerging independence by building the children's confidence, increasing personal responsibility, and gaining problem-solving skills.

Encourage parents to take a copy of the written asthma action plan to the student's school, or childcare or extended care setting, or camp.

Consider the following when selecting treatment options:

- ICSs are the preferred long-term control therapy. The benefits of ICSs outweigh any concerns about potential risks of a small, nonprogressive reduction in growth velocity or other possible adverse effects. ICSs, as with all medications, should be titrated to as low a dose as needed to maintain control. High-quality evidence demonstrates the effectiveness of ICS in children 5–11 years of age, and comparator studies demonstrate improved control with ICS on a range of asthma outcomes compared to other long-term control medications.

- Step up treatment options for children whose asthma is not well controlled on low-dose ICS have not been adequately studied or compared in this age group. The selection will depend on the domain

SAMPLE RECORD FOR MONITORING THE RISK DOMAIN IN CHILDREN: RISK OF ASTHMA PROGRESSION (INCREASED EXACERBATIONS OR NEED FOR DAILY MEDICATION, OR LOSS OF LUNG FUNCTION), AND POTENTIAL ADVERSE EFFECTS OF CORTICOSTEROID THERAPY

Patient name:							
Date							
Long-term control medication							
ICS daily dose*							
LTRA							
LABA							
Theophylline							
Other							
Significant exacerbations							
Exacerbations (number/month)							
Oral systemic corticosteroids (number/year)*							
Hospitalization (number/year)							
Long-term control medication							
Prebronchodilator FEV_1/FVC							
Prebronchodilator FEV_1 percent predicted							
Postbronchodilator FEV_1 percent predicted							
Percent bronchodilator reversibility							
Potential risk of adverse corticosteroid effects (as indicated by corticosteroid dose and duration of treatment)							
Height, cm							
Percentile Plots of growth velocity							

FEV_1, forced expiratory volume in 1 second; FVC, forced vital capacity; ICS, inhaled corticosteroid; LABA, long-acting $beta_2$ agonist; LTRA, leukotriene receptor antagonist

*Consider ophthalmologic exam and bone density measurement in children using high doses of ICS or multiple courses of oral corticosteroids.

of particular relevance (impairment, risk, or both) and clinician–patient preference.

— For the impairment domain:

- Children who have low lung function and >2 days per week impairment may be better served by adding a LABA to a low dose of ICS (based on studies in older children and adults).

- Increasing the dose of ICS to medium dose can improve symptoms and lung function in those children who have greater levels of impairment (based on studies in children).

- One study in children suggests some benefit in the impairment domain with adding LTRA.

— For the risk domain:

- Studies have not demonstrated that adding LABA or LTRA reduces exacerbations in children. Adding LABA has the potential risk of rare life-threatening or fatal exacerbations.

- Studies in older children and adults show that increasing the dose of ICS can reduce the risk of exacerbations, but this may require up to a fourfold increase in the dose. This dose may increase the potential risk of systemic effects, although the risk is small within the medium-dose range.

■ The need for step 4 care usually involves children who have a low level of lung function contributing to their impairment. The combination of ICS and LABA is preferred, on the basis of studies in older children and adults.

■ Before maintenance dose of oral corticosteroids is initiated in step 6, consider a 2-week course of oral corticosteroids to confirm clinical reversibility, measured by spirometry, and the possibility of an effective response to therapy. If the response is poor, a careful review for other pulmonary conditions or comorbid conditions should be conducted to ensure that the primary diagnosis is severe asthma.

Monitor asthma progression. Declines in lung function or repeated periods of worsening asthma impairment may indicate a progressive worsening of the underlying severity of asthma. Although there is no indication that treatment alters the progression of the underlying disease in children, adjustments in treatment may be necessary to maintain asthma control.

Steps for Youths 12 Years of Age and Adults

See figure 16, "Stepwise Approach for Managing Asthma in Youths 12 Years of Age and Adults," for recommended treatment options in different steps and figures 18 and 19, for recommended medication dosages for youths 12 years of age and adults.

Special considerations for this age group include the following:

For youths:

■ Involve adolescents in the development of their written asthma action plans and reviewing their adherence.

■ Encourage students to take a copy of their plan to school, after school programs, and camps.

■ Encourage adolescents to be physically active.

For older adults:

■ Consider a short course of oral systemic corticosteroids to establish reversibility and the extent of possible benefit from asthma treatment. Chronic bronchitis and emphysema may coexist with asthma.

■ Adjust medications as necessary to address coexisting medical conditions. For example, consider calcium and vitamin D supplements for patients who take ICS and have risk factors for osteoporosis. Consider increased sensitivity to side effects of bronchodilators, especially tremor and tachycardia with increasing age, and increased possibilities for drug interactions with theophylline. Consider also that NSAIDs prescribed for arthritis and the beta-blockers prescribed for hypertension or glaucoma may exacerbate asthma.

■ Review the patient's technique and adherence in using medications, and make necessary adjustments. Physical or cognitive impairments may make proper technique difficult.

Consider the following when selecting treatment options:

■ Recommended treatment for step 3 weighs the high-quality evidence demonstrating the benefits of adding LABA to low-dose ICS against the potential risk of rare life-threatening or fatal exacerbations with the use of LABA. The selection will depend on the domain of particular relevance (impairment, risk, or both) and clinician–patient preference.

- Adding LABA more consistently results in improvements in the impairment domain compared to increasing the dose of ICS.
- If the risk domain is of particular concern, then a balance of potential risks needs to be considered.
- Adding LABA to low-dose ICS reduces the frequency of exacerbations to a greater extent than doubling the dose of ICS, but adding LABA has the potential risk of rare life-threatening or fatal exacerbations.
- Increasing the dose of ICS can significantly reduce the risk of exacerbations, but this benefit may require up to a fourfold increase in the ICS dose. This dose may increase the potential risk of systemic effects, although the risk is small within the medium-dose range.

■ Comparator studies demonstrate significantly greater improvements with adding LABA to ICS compared to other adjunctive therapies.

■ Clinicians who administer omalizumab are advised to be prepared and equipped for the identification and treatment of anaphylaxis that may occur, to observe patients for an appropriate period of time following each omalizumab injection (the optimal length of the observation is not established), and to educate patients about the risks of anaphylaxis and how to recognize and treat it if it occurs (e.g., using prescription auto injectors for emergency self treatment, and seeking immediate medical care).

Managing Special Situations

Patients who have asthma may encounter situations that will require adjustments to their asthma management to keep their asthma under control, such as EIB, pregnancy, and surgery.

Exercise-Induced Bronchospasm

EIB should be anticipated in all asthma patients. A history of cough, shortness of breath, chest pain or tightness, wheezing, or endurance problems during exercises suggests EIB. An exercise challenge, in which a 15 percent decrease in PEF or FEV_1 (measured before and after exercise at 5-minute intervals for 20–30 minutes) will establish the diagnosis.

An important dimension of adequate asthma control is a patient's ability to participate in any activity he or she chooses without experiencing asthma symptoms. EIB should not limit either participation or success in vigorous activities.

Recommended treatments for EIB include:

■ **Long-term control therapy, if appropriate.** Frequent or severe EIB may indicate the need to initiate or step up long-term control medications.

■ **Pretreatment before exercise:**

- Inhaled $beta_2$-agonists will prevent EIB for more than 80 percent of patients. SABA used shortly before exercise may be helpful for 2–3 hours. LABA can be protective up to 12 hours, but there is some shortening of the duration of protection when LABA is used on a daily basis. Frequent or chronic use of LABA as pretreatment for EIB is discouraged, as it may disguise poorly controlled persistent asthma.
- LTRAs, with an onset of action generally hours after administration, can attenuate EIB in up to 50 percent of patients.
- Cromolyn or nedocromil taken shortly before exercise is an alternative treatment, but it is not as effective as SABAs.
- A warmup period before exercise may reduce the degree of EIB.
- A mask or scarf over the mouth may attenuate cold-induced EIB.

Pregnancy

Maintaining asthma control during pregnancy is important for the health and well-being of both the mother and her baby. Maintaining lung function is important to ensure oxygen supply to the fetus. Uncontrolled asthma increases the risk of perinatal mortality, preeclampsia, preterm birth, and low-birth-weight infants. It is safer for pregnant women to be treated with asthma medications than to have asthma symptoms and exacerbations.

■ **Monitor the level of asthma control and lung function during prenatal visits.** The course of asthma improves in one-third of women and worsens for one-third of women during pregnancy. Monthly evaluations of asthma will allow the opportunity to step up therapy if necessary and to step down therapy if possible.

- **Albuterol is the preferred SABA.** The most data related to safety during human pregnancy are available for abuterol.

- **ICSs are the preferred long-term control medication. Budesonide is the preferred ICS** because more data are available on using budesonide in pregnant women than are available on other ICSs, and the data are reassuring. However, no data indicate that the other ICS preparations are unsafe during pregnancy.

Surgery

Patients who have asthma are at risk for complications during and after surgery. These complications include acute bronchoconstriction triggered by intubation, hypoxemia and possible hypercapnia, impaired effectiveness of cough, atelectasis, and respiratory infection, and, if a history of sensitivity is present, reactions to latex exposure or some anesthetic agents.

The following actions are recommended to reduce the risk of complications during surgery:

- Before surgery, review the level of asthma control, medication use (especially oral systemic corticosteroids within the past 6 months), and pulmonary function.

- Provide medications before surgery to improve lung function if lung function is not well controlled. A short course of oral systemic corti costeroids may be necessary.

- For patients receiving oral systemic corticosteroids during the 6 months prior to surgery and for selected patients on long-term high-dose ICS, give 100 mg hydrocortisone every 8 hours intravenously during the surgical period, and reduce the dose rapidly within 24 hours after surgery.

Disparities

Multiple factors contribute to the higher rates of poorly controlled asthma and asthma deaths among Blacks and Latinos compared to Whites. These factors include socioeconomic disparities in access to quality medical care, underprescription and underutilization of long-term control medication, cultural beliefs and practices about asthma management, and perhaps biological and pathophysiological differences that affect the underlying severity of asthma and response to treatment. **Heightened awareness of disparities and cultural barriers, improving access to quality care, and improving communication strategies between clinicians and ethnic or racial minority patients regarding use of asthma medications may improve asthma outcomes.**

FIGURE 11. CLASSIFYING ASTHMA SEVERITY AND INITIATING THERAPY IN CHILDREN

Classifying Asthma Severity and Initiating Therapy in Children

Components of Severity		Intermittent		Persistent — Mild		Persistent — Moderate		Persistent — Severe	
		Ages 0–4	Ages 5–11	Ages 0–4	Ages 5–11	Ages 0–4	Ages 5–11	Ages 0–4	Ages 5–11
Impairment	Symptoms	≤2 days/week	≤2 days/week	>2 days/week but not daily	>2 days/week but not daily	Daily	Daily	Throughout the day	Throughout the day
	Nighttime awakenings	0	≤2×/month	1–2×/month	3–4×/month	3–4×/month	>1×/week but not nightly	>1×/week	Often 7×/week
	Short-acting beta₂-agonist use for symptom control	≤2 days/week	≤2 days/week	>2 days/week but not daily	>2 days/week but not daily	Daily	Daily	Several times per day	Several times per day
	Interference with normal activity	None	None	Minor limitation	Minor limitation	Some limitation	Some limitation	Extremely limited	Extremely limited
	Lung Function — FEV₁ (predicted) or peak flow (personal best)	N/A	normal FEV₁ between exacerbations; >80%	N/A	>80%	N/A	60–80%	N/A	<60%
	FEV₁/FVC	N/A	>85%	N/A	>80%	N/A	75–80%	N/A	<75%
Risk	Exacerbations requiring oral systemic corticosteroids (consider severity and interval since last exacerbation)	0–1/year (see notes)	0–1/year (see notes)	≥2 exacerbations in 6 months requiring oral systemic corticosteroids, or ≥4 wheezing episodes/1 year lasting >1 day AND risk factors for persistent asthma	≥2×/year (see notes) Relative annual risk may be related to FEV₁				
Recommended Step for Initiating Therapy (See "Stepwise Approach for Managing Asthma" for treatment steps.) The stepwise approach is meant to assist, not replace, the clinical decisionmaking required to meet individual patient needs.		Step 1 (for both age groups)		Step 2 (for both age groups)		Step 3 and consider short course of oral systemic corticosteroids	Step 3: medium-dose ICS option and consider short course of oral systemic corticosteroids	Step 3 and consider short course of oral systemic corticosteroids	Step 3: medium-dose ICS option OR step 4 and consider short course of oral systemic corticosteroids

In 2–6 weeks, depending on severity, evaluate level of asthma control that is achieved.
- Children 0–4 years old: If no clear benefit is observed in 4–6 weeks, stop treatment and consider alternative diagnoses or adjusting therapy.
- Children 5–11 years old: Adjust therapy accordingly.

Key: FEV₁, forced expiratory volume in 1 second; FVC, forced vital capacity; ICS, inhaled corticosteroids; ICU, intensive care unit; N/A, not applicable

Notes:
- Level of severity is determined by both impairment and risk. Assess impairment domain by caregiver's recall of previous 2–4 weeks. Assign severity to the most severe category in which any feature occurs.
- Frequency and severity of exacerbations may fluctuate over time for patients in any severity category. At present, there are inadequate data to correspond frequencies of exacerbations with different levels of asthma severity. In general, more frequent and severe exacerbations (e.g., requiring urgent, unscheduled care, hospitalization, or ICU admission) indicate greater underlying disease severity. For treatment purposes, patients with ≥2 exacerbations described above may be considered the same as patients who have persistent asthma, even in the absence of impairment levels consistent with persistent asthma.

FIGURE 12. ASSESSING ASTHMA CONTROL AND ADJUSTING THERAPY IN CHILDREN

Key: EIB, exercise-induced bronchospasm; FEV_1, forced expiratory volume in 1 second; FVC, forced vital capacity; ICU, intensive care unit; N/A, not applicable

Notes:

- The level of control is based on the most severe impairment or risk category. Assess impairment domain by patient's or caregiver's recall of previous 2–4 weeks. Symptom assessment for longer periods should reflect a global assessment, such as whether the patient's asthma is better or worse since the last visit.
- At present, there are inadequate data to correspond frequencies of exacerbations with different levels of asthma control. In general, more frequent and intense exacerbations (e.g., requiring urgent, unscheduled care, hospitalization, or ICU admission) indicate poorer disease control.

Assessing Asthma Control and Adjusting Therapy in Children

Components of Control		Well Controlled		Not Well Controlled		Very Poorly Controlled	
		Ages 0–4	Ages 5–11	Ages 0–4	Ages 5–11	Ages 0–4	Ages 5–11
Impairment	Symptoms	≤2 days/week but not more than once on each day		>2 days/week or multiple times on ≤2 days/week		Throughout the day	
	Nighttime awakenings	≤1x/month		>1x/month	≥2x/month	>1x/week	≥2x/week
	Interference with normal activity	None		Some limitation		Extremely limited	
	Short-acting beta₂-agonist use for symptom control (not prevention of EIB)	≤2 days/week		>2 days/week		Several times per day	
	Lung function • FEV_1 (predicted) or peak flow personal best • FEV_1/FVC	N/A	>80% >80%	N/A	60–80% 75–80%	N/A	<60% <75%
Risk	Exacerbations requiring oral systemic corticosteroids	0–1x/year		2–3x/year	≥2x/year	>3x/year	≥2x/year
	Reduction in lung growth	N/A	Requires long-term followup	N/A		N/A	
	Treatment-related adverse effects	Medication side effects can vary in intensity from none to very troublesome and worrisome. The level of intensity does not correlate to specific levels of control but should be considered in the overall assessment of risk.					
Recommended Action for Treatment (See "Stepwise Approach for Managing Asthma" for treatment steps.) The stepwise approach is meant to assist, not replace, clinical decisionmaking required to meet individual patient needs.		• Maintain current step. • Regular followup every 1–6 months. • Consider step down if well controlled for at least 3 months.		Step up 1 step	Step up at least 1 step	• Consider short course of oral systemic corticosteroids. • Step up 1–2 steps	
				Before step up: • Review adherence to medication, inhaler technique, and environmental control. • If alternative treatment was used, discontinue it and use preferred treatment for that step. • Reevaluate the level of asthma control in 2–6 weeks to achieve control; every 1–6 months to maintain control. Children 0–4 years old: If no clear benefit is observed in 4–6 weeks, consider alternative diagnoses or adjusting therapy. Children 5–11 years old: Adjust therapy accordingly. • For side effects, consider alternative treatment options.					

Managing Asthma Long Term

FIGURE 13. STEPWISE APPROACH FOR MANAGING ASTHMA LONG TERM IN CHILDREN, 0–4 YEARS OF AGE AND 5–11 YEARS OF AGE

Step up if needed (first check inhaler technique, adherence, environmental control, and comorbid conditions)

Assess control

Step down if possible (and asthma is well controlled at least 3 months)

Children 0–4 Years of Age

	Intermittent Asthma	Persistent Asthma: Daily Medication				
	Step 1	Step 2	Step 3	Step 4	Step 5	Step 6
			Consult with asthma specialist if step 3 care or higher is required. Consider consultation at step 2.			
Preferred	SABA PRN	Low-dose ICS	Medium-dose ICS	Medium-dose ICS + LABA or Montelukast	High-dose ICS + LABA or Montelukast	High-dose ICS + LABA or Montelukast + Oral corticosteroids
Alternative		Cromolyn or Montelukast				

Each Step: Patient Education and Environmental Control

- SABA as needed for symptoms; intensity of treatment depends on severity of symptoms
- With viral respiratory symptoms: SABA q 4–6 hours up to 24 hours (longer with physician consult). Consider short course of oral systemic corticosteroids if exacerbation is severe or patient has history of previous severe exacerbations.

Caution: Frequent use of SABA may indicate the need to step up treatment. See text for recommendations on initiating daily long-term-control therapy.

Children 5–11 Years of Age

	Intermittent Asthma	Persistent Asthma: Daily Medication				
	Step 1	Step 2	Step 3	Step 4	Step 5	Step 6
			Consult with asthma specialist if step 4 care or higher is required. Consider consultation at step 3.			
Preferred	SABA PRN	Low-dose ICS	Low-dose ICS + LABA, LTRA, or Theophylline OR Medium-dose ICS	Medium-dose ICS + LABA	High-dose ICS + LABA	High-dose ICS + LABA + Oral corticosteroids
Alternative		Cromolyn, LTRA, Nedocromil, or Theophylline		Medium-dose ICS + LTRA or Theophylline	High-dose ICS + LTRA or Theophylline	High-dose ICS + LTRA or Theophylline + oral corticosteroids

Each Step: Patient Education, Environmental Control, and Management of Comorbidities

Steps 2–4: Consider subcutaneous allergen immunotherapy for patients who have persistent, allergic asthma.

Quick-Relief Medication
- SABA as needed for symptoms. Intensity of treatment depends on severity of symptoms: up to 3 treatments at 20-minute intervals as needed. Short course of oral systemic corticosteroids may be needed.

Caution: Increasing use of SABA or use >2 days a week for symptom relief (not prevention of EIB) generally indicates inadequate control and the need to step up treatment.

Notes (Children 0–4 Years of Age)

- The stepwise approach is meant to assist, not replace, the clinical decisionmaking required to meet individual patient needs.
- If an alternative treatment is used and response is inadequate, discontinue it and use the preferred treatment before stepping up.
- If clear benefit is not observed within 4–6 weeks, and patient's/family's medication technique and adherence are satisfactory, consider adjusting therapy or an alternative diagnosis.
- Studies on children 0–4 years of age are limited. Step 2 preferred therapy is based on Evidence A. All other recommendations are based on expert opinion and extrapolation from studies in older children.
- Clinicians who administer immunotherapy should be prepared and equipped to identify and treat anaphylaxis that may occur.

Key: Alphabetical listing is used when more than one treatment option is listed within either preferred or alternative therapy. ICS, inhaled corticosteroid; LABA, inhaled long-acting beta₂-agonist; LTRA, leukotriene receptor antagonist; oral corticosteroids; SABA, inhaled short-acting beta₂-agonist

Notes (Children 5–11 Years of Age)

- The stepwise approach is meant to assist, not replace, the clinical decisionmaking required to meet individual patient needs.
- If an alternative treatment is used and response is inadequate, discontinue it and use the preferred treatment before stepping up.
- Theophylline is a less desirable alternative due to the need to monitor serum concentration levels.
- Steps 1 and 2 medications are based on Evidence A. Step 3 ICS and ICS plus adjunctive therapy are based on Evidence B for efficacy of each treatment and extrapolation from comparator trials in older children and adults—comparator trials are not available for this age group; steps 4–6 are based on expert opinion and extrapolation from studies in older children and adults.
- Immunotherapy for steps 2–4 is based on Evidence B for house-dust mites, animal danders, and pollens; evidence is weak or lacking for molds and cockroaches. Evidence is strongest for immunotherapy with single allergens. The role of allergy in asthma is greater in children than adults.
- Clinicians who administer immunotherapy should be prepared and equipped to identify and treat anaphylaxis that may occur.

Key: Alphabetical listing is used when more than one treatment option is listed within either preferred or alternative therapy. ICS, inhaled corticosteroid; LABA, inhaled long-acting beta₂-agonist; LTRA, leukotriene receptor antagonist; SABA, inhaled short-acting beta₂-agonist

FIGURE 14. CLASSIFYING ASTHMA SEVERITY AND INITIATING TREATMENT IN YOUTHS 12 YEARS OF AGE AND ADULTS

Assessing severity and initiating treatment for patients who are not currently taking long-term control medications

Classification of Asthma Severity ≥12 years of age

Components of Severity		Intermittent	Mild	Moderate	Severe
Impairment Normal FEV_1/FVC: 8–19 yr 85% 20–39 yr 80% 40–59 yr 75% 60–80 yr 70%	Symptoms	≤2 days/week	>2 days/week but not daily	Daily	Throughout the day
	Nighttime awakenings	≤2x/month	3–4x/month	>1x/week but not nightly	Often 7x/week
	Short-acting beta$_2$-agonist use for symptom control (not prevention of EIB)	≤2 days/week	>2 days/week but not daily, and not more than 1x on any day	Daily	Several times per day
	Interference with normal activity	None	Minor limitation	Some limitation	Extremely limited
	Lung function	• Normal FEV_1 between exacerbations • FEV_1 >80% predicted • FEV_1/FVC normal	• FEV_1 ≥80% predicted • FEV_1/FVC normal	• FEV_1 >60% but <80% predicted • FEV_1/FVC reduced 5%	• FEV_1 <60% predicted • FEV_1/FVC reduced >5%
Risk	Exacerbations requiring oral systemic corticosteroids	0–1/year (see note)	≥2/year (see note)		
		Consider severity and interval since last exacerbation. Frequency and severity may fluctuate over time for patients in any severity category. Relative annual risk of exacerbations may be related to FEV_1.			
Recommended Step for Initiating Treatment (See "Stepwise Approach for Managing Asthma" for treatment steps.)		Step 1	Step 2	Step 3 and consider short course of oral systemic corticosteroids	Step 4 or 5
		In 2–6 weeks, evaluate level of asthma control that is achieved and adjust therapy accordingly.			

Key: EIB, exercise-induced bronchospasm; FEV1, forced expiratory volume in 1 second; FVC, forced vital capacity; ICU, intensive care unit

Notes:

- The stepwise approach is meant to assist, not replace, the clinical decisionmaking required to meet individual patient needs.
- Level of severity is determined by assessment of both impairment and risk. Assess impairment domain by patient's/caregiver's recall of previous 2–4 weeks and spirometry. Assign severity to the most severe category in which any feature occurs.
- At present, there are inadequate data to correspond frequencies of exacerbations with different levels of asthma severity. In general, more frequent and intense exacerbations (e.g., requiring urgent, unscheduled care, hospitalization, or ICU admission) indicate greater underlying disease severity. For treatment purposes, patients who had ≥2 exacerbations requiring oral systemic corticosteroids in the past year may be considered the same as patients who have persistent asthma, even in the absence of impairment levels consistent with persistent asthma.

Managing Asthma Long Term

FIGURE 15. ASSESSING ASTHMA CONTROL AND ADJUSTING THERAPY IN YOUTHS ≥12 YEARS OF AGE AND ADULTS

Components of Control		Classification of Asthma Control (≥12 years of age)		
		Well Controlled	**Not Well Controlled**	**Very Poorly Controlled**
Impairment	Symptoms	≤2 days/week	>2 days/week	Throughout the day
	Nighttime awakenings	≤2x/month	1–3x/week	≥4x/week
	Interference with normal activity	None	Some limitation	Extremely limited
	Short-acting beta$_2$-agonist use for symptom control (not prevention of EIB)	≤2 days/week	>2 days/week	Several times per day
	FEV$_1$ or peak flow	>80% predicted/personal best	60–80% predicted/personal best	<60% predicted/personal best
	Validated questionnaires ATAQ ACQ ACT	0 ≤0.75* ≥20	1–2 ≥1.5 16–19	3–4 N/A ≤15
Risk	Exacerbations requiring oral systemic corticosteroids	0–1/year	≥2/year (see note)	≥2/year (see note)
			Consider severity and interval since last exacerbation	
	Progressive loss of lung function	Evaluation requires long-term followup care.		
	Treatment-related adverse effects	Medication side effects can vary in intensity from none to very troublesome and worrisome. The level of intensity does not correlate to specific levels of control but should be considered in the overall assessment of risk.		
Recommended Action for Treatment (See "Stepwise Approach for Managing Asthma" for treatment steps.)		• Maintain current step. • Regular followup at every 1–6 months to maintain control. • Consider step down if well controlled for at least 3 months.	• Step up 1 step. • Reevaluate in 2–6 weeks. • For side effects, consider alternative treatment options.	• Consider short course of oral systemic corticosteroids. • Step up 1–2 steps. • Reevaluate in 2 weeks. • For side effects, consider alternative treatment options.

*ACQ values of 0.76–1.4 are indeterminate regarding well-controlled asthma.

Key: EIB, exercise-induced bronchospasm; ICU, intensive care unit

Notes:

- The stepwise approach is meant to assist, not replace, the clinical decisionmaking required to meet individual patient needs.
- The level of control is based on the most severe impairment or risk category. Assess impairment domain by patient's recall of previous 2–4 weeks and by spirometry/or peak flow measures. Symptom assessment for longer periods should reflect a global assessment, such as inquiring whether the patient's asthma is better or worse since the last visit.
- At present, there are inadequate data to correspond frequencies of exacerbations with different levels of asthma control. In general, more frequent and intense exacerbations (e.g., requiring urgent, unscheduled care, hospitalization, or ICU admission) indicate poorer disease control. For treatment purposes, patients who had ≥2 exacerbations requiring oral systemic corticosteroids in the past year may be considered the same as patients who have not-well-controlled asthma, even in the absence of impairment levels consistent with not-well-controlled asthma.

ATAQ = Asthma Therapy Assessment Questionnaire©
ACQ = Asthma Control Questionnaire©
ACT = Asthma Control Test™
Minimal Important Difference: 1.0 for the ATAQ; 0.5 for the ACQ; not determined for the ACT.

Before step up in therapy:

— Review adherence to medication, inhaler technique, environmental control, and comorbid conditions.

— If an alternative treatment option was used in a step, discontinue and use the preferred treatment for that step.

FIGURE 16. STEPWISE APPROACH FOR MANAGING ASTHMA IN YOUTHS ≥12 YEARS OF AGE AND ADULTS

Intermittent Asthma

Step 1
Preferred:
SABA PRN

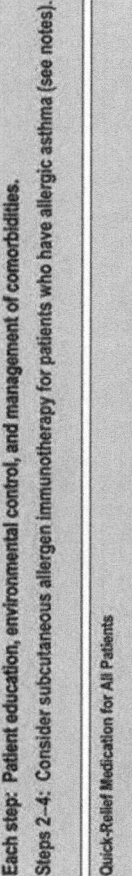

Persistent Asthma: Daily Medication
Consult with asthma specialist if step 4 care or higher is required.
Consider consultation at step 3.

Step 2
Preferred:
Low-dose ICS
Alternative:
Cromolyn, LTRA, Nedocromil, or Theophylline

Step 3
Preferred:
Low-dose ICS + LABA
OR
Medium-dose ICS
Alternative:
Low-dose ICS + either LTRA, Theophylline, or Zileuton

Step 4
Preferred:
Medium-dose ICS + LABA
Alternative:
Medium-dose ICS + either LTRA, Theophylline, or Zileuton

Step 5
Preferred:
High-dose ICS + LABA
AND
Consider Omalizumab for patients who have allergies

Step 6
Preferred:
High-dose ICS + LABA + oral corticosteroid
AND
Consider Omalizumab for patients who have allergies

Step up if needed
(first, check adherence, environmental control, and comorbid conditions)

Assess control

Step down if possible
(and asthma is well controlled at least 3 months)

Each step: Patient education, environmental control, and management of comorbidities.
Steps 2–4: Consider subcutaneous allergen immunotherapy for patients who have allergic asthma (see notes).

Quick-Relief Medication for All Patients
- SABA as needed for symptoms. Intensity of treatment depends on severity of symptoms: up to 3 treatments at 20-minute intervals as needed. Short course of oral systemic corticosteroids may be needed.
- Use of SABA >2 days a week for symptom relief (not prevention of EIB) generally indicates inadequate control and the need to step up treatment.

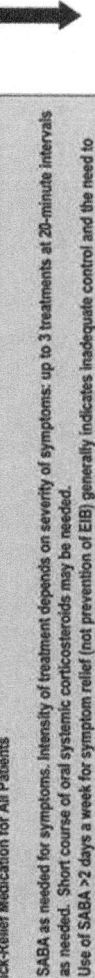

Key: **Alphabetical order is used when more than one treatment option is listed within either preferred or alternative therapy.** ICS, inhaled corticosteroid; LABA, long-acting inhaled beta$_2$-agonist; LTRA, leukotriene receptor antagonist; SABA, inhaled short-acting beta$_2$-agonist

Notes:
- The stepwise approach is meant to assist, not replace, the clinical decisionmaking required to meet individual patient needs.
- If alternative treatment is used and response is inadequate, discontinue it and use the preferred treatment before stepping up.
- Zileuton is a less desirable alternative due to limited studies as adjunctive therapy and the need to monitor liver function. Theophylline requires monitoring of serum concentration levels.
- In step 6, before oral corticosteroids are introduced, a trial of high-dose ICS + LABA + either LTRA, theophylline, or zileuton may be considered, although this approach has not been studied in clinical trials.
- Step 1, 2, and 3 preferred therapies are based on Evidence A; step 3 alternative therapy is based on Evidence A for LTRA, Evidence B for theophylline, and Evidence D for zileuton. Step 4 preferred therapy is based on Evidence B, and alternative therapy is based on Evidence B for LTRA and theophylline and Evidence D zileuton. Step 5 preferred therapy is based on Evidence B. Step 6 preferred therapy is based on (EPR—2 1997) and Evidence B for omalizumab.
- Immunotherapy for steps 2–4 is based on Evidence B for house-dust mites, animal danders, and pollens; evidence is weak or lacking for molds and cockroaches. Evidence is strongest for immunotherapy with single allergens. The role of allergy in asthma is greater in children than in adults.
- Clinicians who administer immunotherapy or omalizumab should be prepared and equipped to identify and treat anaphylaxis that may occur.

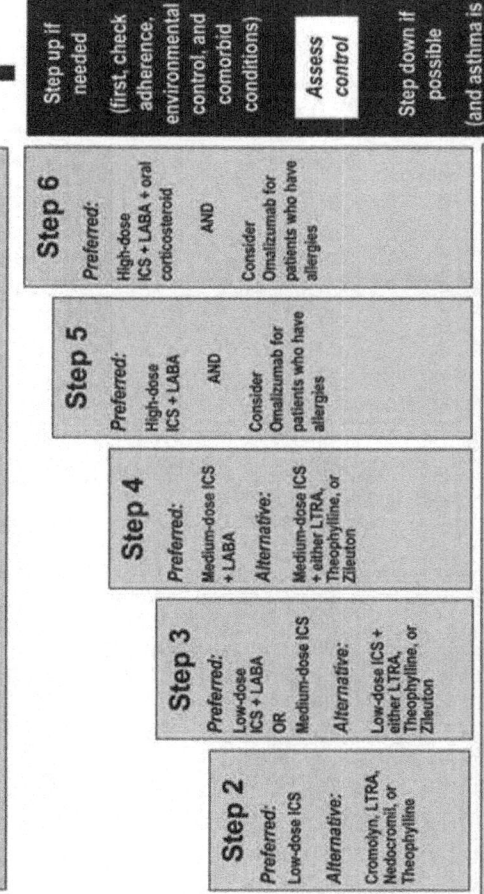

FIGURE 17. USUAL DOSAGES FOR LONG-TERM CONTROL MEDICATIONS*

Medication	0–4 Years of Age	5–11 Years of Age	≥12 Years of Age and Adults	Potential Adverse Effects	Comments (not all inclusive)
Inhaled Corticosteroids (See Figure 18, "Estimated Comparative Daily Dosages for ICSs.")					
Oral Systemic Corticosteroids					(Apply to all three corticosteriods.)
Methylprednisolone 2, 4, 8, 16, 32 mg tablets Prednisolone 5 mg tablets, 5 mg/5 cc, 15 mg/5 cc Prednisone 1, 2.5, 5, 10, 20, 50 mg tablets; 5 mg/cc, 5 mg/5 cc	0.25–2 mg/kg daily in single dose in a.m. or qod as needed for control Short-course "burst": 1–2 mg/kg/day, maximum 60 mg/day for 3–10 days	0.25–2 mg/kg daily in single dose in a.m. or qod as needed for control Short-course "burst": 1–2 mg/kg/day, maximum 60 mg/day for 3–10 days	7.5–60 mg daily in a single dose in a.m. or qod as needed for control Short-course "burst": to achieve control, 40–60 mg per day as single or 2 divided doses for 3–10 days	■ Short-term use: reversible abnormalities in glucose metabolism, increased appetite, fluid retention, weight gain, mood alteration, hypertension, peptic ulcer, and rarely aseptic necrosis. ■ Long-term use: adrenal axis suppression, growth suppression, dermal thinning, hypertension, diabetes, Cushing's syndrome, cataracts, muscle weakness, and—in rare instances—impaired immune function. ■ Consideration should be given to coexisting conditions that could be worsened by systemic corticosteroids, such as herpes virus infections, varicella, tuberculosis, hypertension, peptic ulcer, diabetes mellitus, osteoporosis, and Strongyloides	■ For long-term treatment of severe persistent asthma, administer single dose in a.m. either daily or on alternate days (alternate-day therapy may produce less adrenal suppression). ■ Short courses or "bursts" are effective for establishing control when initiating therapy or during a period of gradual deterioration. ■ There is no evidence that tapering the dose following improvement in symptom control and pulmonary function prevents relapse. ■ Children receiving the lower dose (1 mg/kg/day) experience fewer behavioral side effects, and it appears to be equally efficacious. ■ For patients unable to tolerate the liquid preparations, dexamethasone syrup at 0.4 mg/kg/day may be an alternative. Studies are limited, however, and the longer duration of activity increases the risk of adrenal suppression.
Inhaled Long-Acting Beta$_2$-Agonists (LABAs)					(Apply to both LABAs.)
Salmeterol DPI 50 mcg/blister Formoterol DPI 12 mcg/single-use capsule	NA NA	1 blister q 12 hours 1 capsule q 12 hours	1 blister q 12 hours 1 capsule q 12 hours	■ Tachycardia, skeletal muscle tremor, hypokalemia, prolongation of QTc interval in overdose. ■ A diminished bronchoprotective effect may occur within 1 week of chronic therapy. Clinical significance has not been established. ■ Potential risk of uncommon, severe, life-threatening or fatal exacerbation; see text for additional discussion regarding safety of LABAs.	■ **Should not be used for acute symptom relief or exacerbations. Use only with ICSs.** ■ Decreased duration of protection against EIB may occur with redgular use. ■ Most children <4 years of age cannot provide sufficient inspiratory flow for adequate lung delivery. ■ Do not blow into inhaler after dose is activated. ■ Each capsule is for single use only; additional doses should not be administered for at least 12 hours. ■ Capsules should be used only with the inhaler and should not be taken orally.

Key: DPI, dry powder inhaler; EIB, exercise-induced broncospasm; HFA, hydrofluoroalkane; ICS, inhaled corticosteroids; IgE, immunoglobulin E; MDI, metered-dose inhaler; NA, not available (either not approved, no data available, or safety and efficacy not established for this age group); SABA, short-acting beta$_2$-agonist

*Note: Dosages are provided for those products that have been approved by the U.S. Food and Drug Administration or have sufficient clinical trial safety and efficacy data in the appropriate age ranges to support their use.

FIGURE 17. USUAL DOSAGES FOR LONG-TERM CONTROL MEDICATIONS* (continued)

Medication	0–4 Years of Age	5–11 Years of Age	≥12 Years of Age and Adults	Potential Adverse Effects	Comments (not all inclusive)
Combined Medication					
Fluticasone/Salmeterol DPI 100 mcg/50 mcg, 250 mcg/50 mcg, or 500 mcg/ 50 mcg HFA 45 mcg/21 mcg 115 mcg/21 mcg 230 mcg/21 mcg	NA	1 inhalation bid, dose depends on level of severity or control	1 inhalation bid; dose depends on level of severity or control	■ See notes for ICS and LABA.	■ There have been no clinical trials in children <4 years of age. ■ Most children <4 years of age cannot provide sufficient inspiratory flow for adequate lung delivery. ■ Do not blow into inhaler after dose is activated. ■ 100/50 DPI or 45/21 HFA for patients who have asthma not controlled on low- to medium-dose ICS ■ 250/50 DPI or 115/21 HFA for patients who have asthma not controlled on medium to high dose ICS.
Budesonide/ Formoterol HFA MDI 80 mcg/4.5 mcg 160mcg/4.5 mcg	NA	2 puffs bid, dose depends on level of severity or control	2 puffs bid; dose depends on level of severity or control	■ See notes for ICS and LABA.	■ There have been no clinical trials in children <4 years of age. ■ Currently approved for use in youths ≥12 years of age. Dose for children 5–12 years of age based on clinical trials using DPI with slightly different delivery characteristics. ■ 80/4.5 for patients who have asthma not controlled on low- to medium-dose ICS. ■ 160/4.5 for patients who have asthma not controlled on medium- to high-dose ICS.
Cromolyn/Nedocromil					
Cromolyn MDI 0.8 mg/puff Nebulizer 20 mg/ampule Nedocromil MDI 1.75 mg/puff	NA 1 ampule qid NA <2 years of age NA <6 years of age	2 puffs qid 1 ampule qid 2 puffs qid	2 puffs qid 1 ampule qid 2 puffs qid	■ Cough and irritation. ■ 15–20 percent of patients complain of an unpleasant taste from nedocromil. ■ Safety is the primary advantage of these	■ One dose of cromolyn before exercise or allergen exposure provides effective prophylaxis for 1–2 hours. Not as effective as inhaled beta$_2$-agonists for EIB as SABA. ■ 4- to 6-week trial of cromolyn or nedocromil may be needed to determine maximum benefit. ■ Dose by MDI may be inadequate to affect hyperresponsiveness. ■ Once control is achieved, the frequency of dosing may be reduced.

Managing Asthma Long Term

FIGURE 17. USUAL DOSAGES FOR LONG-TERM CONTROL MEDICATIONS* (continued)

Medication	0–4 Years of Age	5–11 Years of Age	≥12 Years of Age and Adults	Potential Adverse Effects	Comments (not all inclusive)
Immunomodulators					
Omalizumab (Anti IgE) Subcutaneous injection, 150 mg/1.2 mL following reconstitution with 1.4 mL sterile water for injection	NA	NA	150–375 mg SC q 2–4 weeks, depending on body weight and pretreatment serum IgE level	■ Pain and bruising of injection sites in 5–20 percent of patients. ■ Anaphylaxis has been reported in 0.2% of treated patients. ■ Malignant neoplasms were reported in 0.5 percent of patients compared to 0.2 percent receiving placebo; relationship to drug is unclear.	■ Do not administer more than 150 mg per injection site. ■ Monitor patients following injections; be prepared and equipped to identify and treat anaphylaxis that may occur. ■ Whether patients will develop significant antibody titers to the drug with long-term administration is unknown.
Leukotriene Modifiers					
Leukotriene Receptor Antagonists (LTRAs) Montelukast 4 mg or 5 mg chewable tablet 4 mg granule packets 10 mg tablet	4 mg qhs (1–5 years of age)	5 mg qhs (6–14 years of age)	10 mg qhs	■ No specific adverse effects have been identified. ■ Rare cases of Churg-Strauss have occurred, but the association is unclear.	■ Montelukast exhibits a flat dose-response curve. Doses >10 mg will not produce a greater response in adults. ■ No more efficacious than placebo in infants ages 6–24 months. ■ As long-term therapy may attenuate exercise-induced bronchospasm in some patients, but less effective than ICS therapy.
Zafirlukast 10 mg tablet 20 mg tablet	NA	10 mg bid (7–11 years of age)	40 mg daily (20 mg tablet bid)	■ Postmarketing surveillance has reported cases of reversible hepatitis and, rarely, irreversible hepatic failure resulting in death and liver transplantation.	■ For zafirlukast, administration with meals decreases bioavailability; take at least 1 hour before or 2 hours after meals. ■ Zarfirlukast is a microsomal P450 enzyme inhibitor that can inhibit the metabolism of warfarin. Doses of these drugs should be monitored accordingly. ■ Monitor hepatic enzymes (ALT). Warn patients to discontinue use if they experience signs and symptoms of liver dysfunction.
5-Lipoxygenase Inhibitor Zileuton 600 mg tablet	NA	NA	2,400 mg daily (give tablets qid)	■ Elevation of liver enzymes has been reported. Limited case reports of reversible hepatitis and hyperbilirubinemia.	■ For zileuton, monitor hepatic enzymes (ALT). ■ Zileuton is a microsomal P450 enzyme inhibitor that can inhibit the metabolism of warfarin and theophylline. Doses of these drugs should be monitored accordingly.
Methylxanthines					
Theophylline Liquids, sustained-release tablets, and capsules	Starting dose 10 mg/kg/day; usual maximum: ■ <1 year of age: 0.2 (age in weeks) + 5 = mg/kg/day ■ ≥1 year of age: 16 mg/kg/day	Starting dose 10 mg/kg/day; usual maximum: 16 mg/kg/day	Starting dose 10 mg/kg/day up to 300 mg maximum; usual maximum: 800 mg/day	■ Dose-related acute toxicities include tachycardia, nausea and vomiting, tachyarrhythmias (SVT), central nervous system stimulation, headache, seizures, hematemesis, hyperglycemia, and hypokalemia. ■ Adverse effects at usual therapeutic doses include insomnia, gastric upset, aggravation of ulcer or reflux, increase in hyperactivity in some children, difficulty in urination in elderly males who have prostatism.	■ Adjust dosage to achieve serum concentration of 5–15 mcg/mL at steady state (at least 48 hours on same dosage). ■ Due to wide interpatient variability in theophylline metabolic clearance, routine serum theophylline level monitoring is essential. ■ Patients should be told to discontinue if they experience toxicity. ■ Various factors (diet, food, febrile illness, age, smoking, and other medications) can affect serum concentrations. See EPR—3 Full Report 2007 and package inserts for details.

FIGURE 18. ESTIMATED COMPARATIVE DAILY DOSAGES FOR INHALED CORTICOSTEROIDS

Drug	Low Daily Dose - Child 0–4 Years of Age	Low Daily Dose - Child 5–11 Years of Age	Low Daily Dose - ≥12 Years of Age and Adults	Medium Daily Dose - Child 0–4 Years of Age	Medium Daily Dose - Child 5–11 Years of Age	Medium Daily Dose - ≥12 Years of Age and Adults	High Daily Dose - Child 0–4 Years of Age	High Daily Dose - Child 5–11 Years of Age	High Daily Dose - ≥12 Years of Age and Adults
Beclomethasone HFA 40 or 80 mcg/puff	NA	80–160 mcg	80–240 mcg	NA	>160–320 mcg	>240–480 mcg	NA	>320 mcg	>480 mcg
Budesonide DPI 90, 180, or 200 mcg/inhalation	NA	180–400 mcg	180–600 mcg	NA	>400–800 mcg	>600–1,200 mcg	NA	>800 mcg	>1,200 mcg
Budesonide Inhaled Inhalation suspension for nebulization	0.25–0.5 mg	0.5 mg	NA	>0.5–1.0 mg	1.0 mg	NA	>1.0 mg	2.0 mg	NA
Flunisolide 250 mcg/puff	NA	500–750 mcg	500–1,000 mcg	NA	1,000–1,250 mcg	>1,000–2,000 mcg	NA	>1,250 mcg	>2,000 mcg
Flunisolide HFA 80 mcg/puff	NA	160 mcg	320 mcg	NA	320 mcg	>320–640 mcg	NA	≥640 mcg	>640 mcg
Fluticasone HFA/MDI: 44, 110, or 220 mcg/puff	176 mcg	88–176 mcg	88–264 mcg	>176–352 mcg	>176–352 mcg	>264–440 mcg	>352 mcg	>352 mcg	>440 mcg
DPI: 50, 100, or 250 mcg/inhalation	NA	100–200 mcg	100–300 mcg	NA	>200–400 mcg	>300–500 mcg	NA	>400 mcg	>500 mcg
Mometasone DPI 200 mcg/inhalation	NA	NA	200 mcg	NA	NA	400 mcg	NA	NA	>400 mcg
Triamcinolone acetonide 75 mcg/puff	NA	300–600 mcg	300–750 mcg	NA	>600–900 mcg	>750–1,500 mcg	NA	>900 mcg	>1,500 mcg

Key: DPI, dry power inhaler; HFA, hydrofluoroalkane; MDI, metered-dose inhaler; NA, not available (either not approved, no data available, or safety and efficacy not established for this age group)

Therapeutic Issues:

- The most important determinant of appropriate dosing is the clinician's judgment of the patient's response to therapy. The clinician must monitor the patient's response on several clinical parameters and adjust the dose accordingly. Once control of asthma is achieved, the dose should be carefully titrated to the minimum dose required to maintain control.

- Preparations are not interchangeable on a mcg or per puff basis. This figure presents estimated comparable daily doses. See EPR—3 Full Report 2007 for full discussion.

- Some doses may be outside package labeling, especially in the high-dose range. Budesonide nebulizer suspension is the only inhaled corticosteroid (ICS) with FDA-approved labeling for children <4 years of age.

- For children <4 years of age: The safety and efficacy of ICSs in children <1 year has not been established. Children <4 years of age generally require delivery of ICS (budesonide and fluticasone HFA) through a face mask that should fit snugly over nose and mouth and avoid nebulizing in the eyes. Wash face after each treatment to prevent local corticosteroid side effects. For budesonide, the dose may be administered 1–3 times daily. Budesonide suspension is compatible with albuterol, ipratropium, and levalbuterol nebulizer solutions in the same nebulizer. Use only jet nebulizers, as ultrasonic nebulizers are ineffective for suspensions. For fluticasone HFA, the dose should be divided 2 times daily; the low dose for children <4 years of age is higher than for children 5–11 years of age due to lower dose delivered with face mask and data on efficacy in young children.

Potential Adverse Effects of Inhaled Corticosteroids:

- Cough, dysphonia, oral thrush (candidiasis).

- Spacer or valved holding chamber with non-breath-actuated MDIs and mouthwashing and spitting after inhalation decrease local side effects.

- A number of the ICSs, including fluticasone, budesonide, and mometasone, are metabolized in the gastrointestinal tract and liver by CYP 3A4 isoenzymes. Potent inhibitors of CYP 3A4, such as ritonavir and ketoconazole, have the potential for increasing systemic concentrations of these ICSs by increasing oral availability and decreasing systemic clearance. Some cases of clinically significant Cushing syndrome and secondary adrenal insufficiency have been reported.

- In high doses, systemic effects may occur, although studies are not conclusive, and clinical significance of these effects has not been established (e.g., adrenal suppression, osteoporosis, skin thinning, and easy bruising). In low-to-medium doses, suppression of growth velocity has been observed in children, but this effect may be transient, and the clinical significance has not been established.

FIGURE 19. USUAL DOSAGES FOR QUICK-RELIEF MEDICATIONS*

Medication	<5 Years of Age	5–11 Years of Age	≥12 Years of Age and Adults	Potential Adverse Effects	Comments (not all inclusive)
Inhaled Short-Acting Beta$_2$-Agonists					
	Dose applies to Albuterol.	*Dose applies to Albuterol/and Levalbuterol.*	*Dose applies to all four SABAs*		*Apply to all four (SABAs)*
MDI					
Albuterol CFC 90 mcg/puff, 200 puffs/canister	1–2 puffs 5 minutes before exercise	2 puffs 5 minutes before exercise	2 puffs 5 minutes before exercise	■ Tachycardia, skeletal muscle tremor, hypokalemia, increased lactic acid, headache, hyperglycemia. Inhaled route, in general, causes few systemic adverse effects. Patients with preexisting cardiovascular disease, especially the elderly, may have adverse cardiovascular reactions with inhaled therapy.	■ Drugs of choice for acute bronchospasm. ■ Differences in potencies exist, but all products are essentially comparable on a puff per puff basis. ■ An increasing use or lack of expected effect indicates diminished control of asthma. ■ Not recommended for long-term daily treatment. Regular use exceeding 2 days/week for symptom control (not prevention of EIB) indicates the need for additional long-term control therapy. ■ May double usual dose for mild exacerbations. ■ For levalbuterol, prime the inhaler by releasing 4 actuations prior to use. ■ For HFA: periodically clean HFA actuator, as drug may plug orifice. ■ For autohaler: children <4 years of age may not generate sufficient inspiratory flow to activate an auto-inhaler. ■ Nonselective agents (i.e., epinephrine, isoproterenol, metaproterenol) are not recommended due to their potential for excessive cardiac stimulation, especially in high doses.
Albuterol HFA 90 mcg/puff, 200 puffs/canister	2 puffs every 4–6 hours, as needed for symptoms	2 puffs every 4–6 hours, as needed for symptoms	2 puffs every 4–6 hours, as needed for symptoms		
Levalbuterol HFA 45 mcg/puff, 200 puffs/canister	NA <4 years of age				
Pirbuterol CFC Autohaler 200 mcg/puff, 400 puffs/canister	NA	NA			
Nebulizer solution					■ May mix with cromolyn solution, budesonide inhalant suspension, or ipratropium solution for nebulization. May double dose for severe exacerbations. ■ Does not have FDA-approved labeling for children <6 years of age. ■ Compatible with budesonide inhalant suspension. The product is a sterile-filled preservative-free unit dose vial.
Albuterol 0.63 mg/3 mL 1.25 mg/3 mL 2.5 mg/3 mL 5 mg/mL (0.5%)	0.63–2.5 mg in 3 cc of saline q 4–6 hours, as needed	1.25–5 mg in 3 cc of saline q 4–8 hours, as needed	1.25–5 mg in 3 cc of saline q 4–8 hours, as needed	(Same as with MDI)	
Levalbuterol (R-albuterol) 0.31 mg/3 mL 0.63 mg/3 mL 1.25 mg/0.5 mL 1.25 mg/3 mL	0.31–1.25 mg in 3 cc q 4–6 hours, as needed for symptoms	0.31–0.63 mg, q 8 hours, as needed for symptoms	0.63 mg– 1.25 mg q 8 hours, as needed for symptoms	(Same as with MDI)	

Key: CFC, chlorofluorocarbon; ED, emergency department; EIB, exercise-induced bronchospasm; HFA, hydrofluoroalkane; IM, intramuscular; MDI, metered-dose inhaler; NA, not available (either not approved, no data available, or safety and efficacy not established for this age group); PEF, peak expiratory flor; SABA, short-acting beta$_2$-agonist

*Dosages are provided for those products that have been approved by the U.S. Food and Drug Administration (FDA) or have sufficient clinical trial safety and efficacy data in the appropriate age ranges to support their use.

FIGURE 19. USUAL DOSAGES FOR QUICK-RELIEF MEDICATIONS* (continued)

Medication	<5 Years of Age	5–11 Years of Age	≥12 Years of Age and Adults	Potential Adverse Effects	Comments (not all inclusive)
Anticholinergics					
Ipratropium HFA				Drying of mouth and respiratory secretions, increased wheezing in some individuals, blurred vision if sprayed in eyes. If used in the ED, produces less cardiac stimulation than SABAs.	■ Multiple doses in the emergency department (not hospital) setting provide additive benefit to SABA. ■ Treatment of choice for bronchospasm due to beta-blocker medication. ■ Does not block EIB. ■ Reverses only cholinergically mediated bronchospasm; does not modify reaction to antigen. ■ May be an alternative for patients who do not tolerate SABA. ■ Has not proven to be efficacious as long-term control therapy for asthma.
MDI 17 mcg/puff, 200 puffs/canister	NA	NA	2–3 puffs q 6 hours		
Nebulizer solution 0.25 mg/mL (0.025%)	NA	NA	0.25 mg q 6 hours		
Ipratropium with albuterol					
MDI 18 mcg/puff of ipratropium bromide and 90 mcg/puff of albuterol 200 puffs/canister	NA	NA	2–3 puffs q 6 hours		
Nebulizer solution 0.5 mg/3 mL ipratropium bromide and 2.5 mg/3 mL albuterol	NA	NA	3 mL q 4–6 hours		■ Contains EDTA to prevent discoloration of the solution. This additive does not induce bronchospasm.
Systemic Corticosteroids					
Methylprednisolone 2, 4, 6, 8, 16, 32 mg tablets Prednisolone 5 mg tablets, 5 mg/5 cc, 15 mg/5 cc Prednisone 1, 2.5, 5, 10, 20, 50 mg tablets; 5 mg/cc, 5 mg/5 cc	*Dosages apply to first three corticosteroids.* Short course "burst:" 1–2 mg/kg/day, maximum 60 mg/day, for 3–10 days	Short course "burst": 1–2 mg/kg/day maximum 60 mg/day for 3–10 days	Short course "burst": 40–60 mg/day as single or 2 divided doses for 3–10 days	■ Short-term use: reversible abnormalities in glucose metabolism, increased appetite, fluid retention, weight gain, facial flushing, mood alteration, hypertension, peptic ulcer, and rarely aseptic necrosis. ■ Consideration should be given to coexisting conditions that could be worsened by systemic corticosteroids, such as herpes virus infections, varicella, tuberculosis, hypertension, peptic ulcer, diabetes mellitus, osteoporosis, and *Strongyloides*.	*(Applies to the first three corticosteroids.)* ■ Short courses or "bursts" are effective for establishing control when initiating therapy or during a period of gradual deterioration. Action may begin within an hour. ■ The burst should be continued until patient achieves 80 percent PEF personal best or symptoms resolve. This usually requires 3–10 days but may require longer. There is no evidence that tapering the dose following improvement prevents relapse in asthma exacerbations. ■ Other systemic corticosteroids such as hydrocortisone and dexamethasone given in equipotent daily doses are likely to be as effective as prednisolone.

Managing Asthma Long Term

FIGURE 19. USUAL DOSAGES FOR QUICK-RELIEF MEDICATIONS* (continued)

Medication	<5 Years of Age	5–11 Years of Age	≥12 Years of Age and Adults	Potential Adverse Effects	Comments (not all inclusive)
Systemic Corticosteroids (continued)					
Repository injection (Methylprednisolone acetate) 40 mg/mL 80 mg/mL	7.5 mg/kg IM once	240 mg IM once	240 mg IM once		■ May be used in place of a short burst of oral steroids in patients who are vomiting or if adherence is a problem.

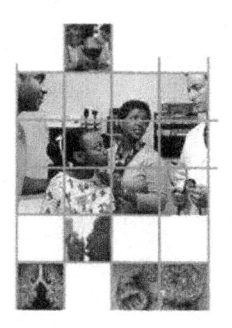

Managing Exacerbations

Asthma exacerbations are acute or subacute episodes of progressively worsening shortness of breath, cough, wheezing, and chest tightness, or some combination of these symptoms. Exacerbations are characterized by decreases in expiratory airflow; objective measures of lung function (spirometry or PEF) are more reliable indicators of severity than symptoms are. Individuals whose asthma is well controlled with ICSs have decreased risk of exacerbations. However, these patients can still be vulnerable to exacerbations, for example, when they have viral respiratory infections.

Effective management of exacerbations incorporates the same four components of asthma management used in managing asthma long term: assessment and monitoring, patient education, environmental control, and medications.

Classifying Severity

Do not underestimate the severity of an exacerbation. Severe exacerbations can be life threatening and can occur in patients at any level of asthma severity—i.e., intermittent, or mild, moderate, or severe persistent asthma. See figure 20, "Classifying Severity of Asthma Exacerbations in the Urgent or Emergency Care Setting."

Patients at high risk of asthma-related death require special attention—particularly intensive education, monitoring, and care. Such patients should be advised to seek medical care early during an exacerbation. Risk factors for asthma-related death include:

- Previous severe exacerbation (e.g., intubation or ICU admission for asthma)
- Two or more hospitalizations or >3 ED visits in the past year
- Use of >2 canisters of SABA per month
- Difficulty perceiving airway obstruction or the severity of worsening asthma
- Low socioeconomic status or inner-city residence
- Illicit drug use
- Major psychosocial problems or psychiatric disease
- Comorbidities, such as cardiovascular disease or other chronic lung disease

Home Management

Early treatment by the patient at home is the best strategy for managing asthma exacerbations. Patients should be instructed how to:

- **Use a written asthma action plan** that notes when and how to treat signs of an exacerbation. A peak flow-based plan may be particularly useful for patients who have difficulty perceiving airflow obstruction or have a history of severe exacerbations.
- **Recognize early indicators of an exacerbation,** including worsening PEF.
- **Adjust their medications** by increasing SABA and, in some cases, adding a short course of oral systemic corticosteroids. Doubling the dose of ICSs is not effective.
- **Remove or withdraw from allergens or irritants** in the environment that may contribute to the exacerbation.
- **Monitor response to treatment and promptly communicate with the clinician about any serious deterioration** in symptoms or PEF or about decreased responsiveness to SABA treatment, including decreased duration of effect.

The following home management techniques are not recommended because no studies demonstrate their effectiveness and they may delay patients from obtaining necessary care: drinking large volumes of liquids; breathing warm, moist air; or using over-the-counter products, such as antihistamines or cold remedies. Pursed-lip and other forms of breathing may help to maintain calm, but these methods do not improve lung function.

FIGURE 20. CLASSIFYING SEVERITY OF ASTHMA EXACERBATIONS IN THE URGENT OR EMERGENCY CARE SETTING

Note: Patients are instructed to use quick-relief medications if symptoms occur or if PEF drops below 80 percent predicted or personal best. If PEF is 50–79 percent, the patient should monitor response to quick-relief medication carefully and consider contacting a clinician. If PEF is below 50 percent, immediate medical care is usually required. In the urgent or emergency care setting, the following parameters describe the severity and likely clinical course of an exacerbation.

	Symptoms and Signs	Initial PEF (or FEV1)	Clinical Course
Mild	Dyspnea only with activity (assess tachypnea in young children)	PEF ≥ 70 percent predicted or personal best	■ Usually cared for at home ■ Prompt relief with inhaled SABA ■ Possible short course of oral systemic corticosteroids
Moderate	Dyspnea interferes with or limits usual activity	PEF 40–69 percent predicted or personal best	■ Usually requires office or ED visit ■ Relief from frequent inhaled SABA ■ Oral systemic corticosteroids; some symptoms last for 1–2 days after treatment is begun
Severe	Dyspnea at rest; interferes with conversation	PEF <40 percent predicted or personal best	■ Usually requires ED visit and likely hospitalization ■ Partial relief from frequent inhaled SABA ■ Oral systemic corticosteroids; some symptoms last for >3 days after treatment is begun ■ Adjunctive therapies are helpful
Subset: Life threatening	Too dyspneic to speak; perspiring	PEF <25 percent predicted or personal best	■ Requires ED/hospitalization; possible ICU ■ Minimal or no relief from frequent inhaled SABA ■ Intravenous corticosteroids ■ Adjunctive therapies are helpful

Key: ED, emergency department; FEV_1, forced expiratory volume in 1 second; ICU, intensive care unit; PEF, peak expiratory flow; SABA, short-acting $beta_2$-agonist

Management in the Urgent or Emergency Care and Hospital Settings

Emergency medical services providers should have prehospital protovols that allow administration of SABA, supplemental oxygen, and (with appropriate medical oversight) anticholinergics and oral systemic corticosteriods to patients who have signs or symptoms of an asthma exacerbation.

Treatment strategies for managing moderate or severe exacerbations in the urgent or emergency care setting are described below. Also see figure 21 for a detailed sequence of recommended actions for monitoring and treatment and figure 22 for dosages of drugs for asthma exacerbations.

- **Administer supplemental oxygen** to correct significant hypoxemia in moderate or severe exacerbations.

- **Administer repetitive or continuous administration of SABA** to reverse airflow obstruction rapidly.

- **Administer oral systemic corticosteroids** to decrease airway inflammation in moderate or severe exacerbations or for patients who fail to respond promptly and completely to SABA treatment.

- **Monitor response to therapy with serial assessments.**

  — For children:

FIGURE 21. MANAGEMENT OF ASTHMA EXACERBATIONS: EMERGENCY DEPARTMENT AND HOSPITAL-BASED CARE

Initial Assessment
Brief history, physical examination (auscultation, use of accessory muscles, heart rate, respiratory rate), PEF or FEV_1, oxygen saturation, and other tests as indicated

FEV_1 or PEF ≥40% (Mild-to-Moderate)
- Oxygen to achieve SaO_2 ≥90%
- Inhaled SABA by nebulizer or MDI with valved holding chamber, up to 3 doses in first hour
- Oral systemic corticosteroids if no immediate response or if patient recently took oral systemic corticosteroids

FEV_1 or PEF <40% (Severe)
- Oxygen to achieve SaO_2 ≥ 90%
- High-dose inhaled SABA plus ipratropium by nebulizer or MDI plus valved holding chamber, every 20 minutes or continuously for 1 hour
- Oral systemic corticosteroids

Impending or Actual Respiratory Arrest
- Intubation and mechanical ventilation with 100% oxygen
- Nebulized SABA and ipratropium
- Intravenous corticosteroids
- Consider adjunct therapies

Admit to Hospital Intensive Care (see box below)

Repeat Assessment
Symptoms, physical examination, PEF, O_2 saturation, other tests as needed

Moderate Exacerbation
FEV_1 or PEF 40–69% predicted/personal best
Physical exam: moderate symptoms
- Inhaled SABA every 60 minutes
- Oral systemic corticosteroid
- Continue treatment 1–3 hours, provided there is improvement; make admit decision in <4 hours

Severe Exacerbation
FEV_1 or PEF <40% predicted/personal best
Physical exam: severe symptoms at rest, accessory muscle use, chest retraction
History: high-risk patient
No improvement after initial treatment
- Oxygen
- Nebulized SABA plus ipratropium, hourly or continuous
- Oral systemic corticosteroids
- Consider adjunct therapies

Good Response
- FEV_1 or PEF ≥70%
- Response sustained 60 minutes after last treatment
- No distress
- Physical exam: normal

Incomplete Response
- FEV_1 or PEF 40–69%
- Mild-to-moderate symptoms

Individualized decision re: hospitalization (see text)

Poor Response
- FEV_1 or PEF <40%
- PCO_2 ≥42 mm Hg
- Physical exam: symptoms severe, drowsiness, confusion

Discharge Home
- Continue treatment with inhaled SABA
- Continue course of oral systemic corticosteroid
- Consider initiation of an ICS
- Patient education
  - Review medications, including inhaler technique
  - Review/initiate action plan
  - Recommend close medical followup

Admit to Hospital Ward
- Oxygen
- Inhaled SABA
- Systemic (oral or intravenous) corticosteroid
- Consider adjunct therapies
- Monitor vital signs, FEV_1 or PEF, SaO_2

Admit to Hospital Intensive Care
- Oxygen
- Inhaled SABA hourly or continuously
- Intravenous corticosteroid
- Consider adjunct therapies
- Possible intubation and mechanical ventilation

Improve

Discharge Home
- Continue treatment with inhaled SABAs.
- Continue course of oral systemic corticosteroid.
- Continue on ICS. For those not on long-term-control therapy, consider initiation of an ICS.
- Patient education (e.g., review medications, including inhaler technique; review/initiate action plan and, whenever possible, environmental control measures; and recommend close medical followup).
- Before discharge, schedule followup appointment with primary care provider and/or asthma specialist in 1–4 weeks.

Key: FEV_1, forced expiratory volume in 1 second; ICS, inhaled corticosteroid; MDI, metered-dose inhaler; PCO2, partial pressure carbon dioxide; PEF, peak expiratory flow; SABA, short-acting beta$_2$-agonist; SaO2, oxygen saturation

FIGURE 22. DOSAGES OF DRUGS FOR ASTHMA EXACERBATIONS

Medication	Child Dose*	Adult Dose	Comments (not all inclusive)
Inhaled Short-Acting Beta$_2$-Agonists (SABA)			
Albuterol Nebulizer solution (0.63 mg/3 mL, 1.25 mg/3 mL, 2.5 mg/3 mL, 5.0 mg/mL)	0.15 mg/kg (minimum dose 2.5 mg) every 20 minutes for 3 doses then 0.15–0.3 mg/kg up to 10 mg every 1–4 hours as needed, or 0.5 mg/kg/hour by continuous nebulization.	2.5–5 mg every 20 minutes for 3 doses, then 2.5–10 mg every 1–4 hours as needed, or 10–15 mg/hour continuously.	Only selective beta$_2$ agonists are recommended. For optimal delivery, dilute aerosols to minimum of 3 mL at gas flow of 6–8 L/min. Use large volume nebulizers for continuous administration. May mix with ipratropium nebulizer solution.
MDI (90 mcg/puff)	4–8 puffs every 20 minutes for 3 doses, then every 1–4 hours inhalation maneuver as needed. Use VHC; add mask in children <4 years.	4–8 puffs every 20 minutes up to 4 hours, then every 1–4 hours as needed.	In mild-to-moderate exacerbations, MDI plus VHC is as effective as nebulized therapy with appropriate administration technique and coaching by trained personnel.
Bitolterol Nebulizer solution (2 mg/mL)	See albuterol dose; thought to be half as potent as albuterol on mg basis.	See albuterol dose.	Has not been studied in severe asthma exacerbations. Do not mix with other drugs.
MDI (370 mcg/puff)	See albuterol MDI dose.	See albuterol MDI dose.	Has not been studied in severe asthma exacerbations.
Levalbuterol (R-albuterol) Nebulizer solution (0.63 mg/3 mL, 1.25 mg/0.5 mL 1.25 mg/3 mL)	0.075 mg/kg (minimum dose 1.25 mg) every 20 minutes for 3 doses, then 0.075–0.15 mg/kg up to 5 mg every 1–4 hours as needed.	1.25–2.5 mg every 20 minutes for 3 doses, then 1.25–5 mg every 1–4 hours as needed.	Levalbuterol administered in one-half the mg dose of albuterol provides comparable efficacy and safety. Has not been evaluated by continuous nebulization.
MDI (45 mcg/puff)	See albuterol MDI dose	See albuterol MDI dose.	
Pirbuterol MDI (200 mcg/puff)	See albuterol MDI dose; thought to be half as potent as albuterol on a mg basis.	See albuterol MDI dose.	Has not been studied in severe asthma exacerbations
Systemic (Injected) Beta$_2$-Agonists			
Epinephrine 1:1,000 (1 mg/mL)	0.01 mg/kg up to 0.3–0.5 mg every 20 minutes for 3 doses sq.	0.3–0.5 mg every 20 minutes for 3 doses sq.	No proven advantage of systemic therapy over aerosol.
Terbutaline (1 mg/mL)	0.01 mg/kg every 20 minutes for 3 doses then every 2–6 hours as needed sq.	0.25 mg every 20 minutes for 3 doses sq.	No proven advantage of systemic therapy over aerosol.
Anticholinergics			
Ipratropium bromide Nebulizer solution (0.25 mg/mL)	0.25–0.5 mg every 20 minutes for 3 doses, then as needed	0.5 mg every 20 minutes for 3 doses, then as needed	May mix in same nebulizer with albuterol. Should not be used as first-line therapy; should be added to SABA therapy for severe exacerbations. The addition of ipratropium has not been shown to provide further benefit once the patient is hospitalized.
MDI (18 mcg/puff)	4–8 puffs every 20 minutes as needed up to 3 hours	8 puffs every 20 minutes as needed up to 3 hours	Should use with VHC and face mask for children <4 years. Studies have examined ipratropium bromide MDI for up to 3 hours.

FIGURE 22. DOSAGES OF DRUGS FOR ASTHMA EXACERBATIONS (continued)

Medication	Child Dose*	Adult Dose	Comments (not all inclusive)
Anticholinergics (continued)			
Ipratropium with albuterol Nebulizer solution (Each 3 mL vial contains 0.5 mg ipratropium bromide and 2.5 mg albuterol.)	1.5-3 mL every 20 minutes for 3 doses, then as needed	3 mL every 20 minutes for 3 doses, then as needed	May be used for up to 3 hours in the initial management of severe exacerbations. The addition of ipratropium to albuterol has not been shown to provide further benefit once the patient is hospitalized.
MDI (Each puff contains 18 mcg ipratropium bromide and 90 mcg of albuterol.)	4–8 puffs every 20 minutes as needed up to 3 hours	8 puffs every 20 minutes as needed up to 3 hours	Should use with VHC and face mask for children <4 years.
Systemic Corticosteroids (Apply to all three corticosteriods.)			
Prednisone Methylprednisolone Prednisolone	1-2 mg/kg in 2 divided doses (maximum = 60 mg/day) until PEF is 70 percent of predicted or personal best	40–80 mg/day in 1 or 2 divided doses until PEF reaches 70 percent of predicted or personal best	For outpatient "burst," use 40–60 mg in single or 2 divided doses for total of 5–10 days in adults (children: 1–2 mg/kg/day maximum 60 mg/day for 3–10 days).

* Children ≤ 12 years of age
Key: ED, emergency department; MDI, metered-dose inhaler; PEF, peak expiratory flow, VHC, valved holding chamber

Notes:
- There is no known advantage for higher doses of corticosteroids in severe asthma exacerbations, nor is there any advantage for intravenous administration over oral therapy provided gastrointestinal transit time or absorption is not impaired.
- The total course of systemic corticosteroids for an asthma exacerbation requiring an ED visit of hospitalization may last from 3 to 10 days. For corticosteroid courses of less than 1 week, there is no need to taper the dose. For slightly longer courses (e.g., up to 10 days), there probably is no need to taper, especially if patients are concurrently taking ICSs.
- ICSs can be started at any point in the treatment of an asthma exacerbation.

- No single measure is best for assessing severity or predicting hospital admission.
- Lung function measures (FEV_1 or PEF) may be useful for children ≥5 years of age, but these measures may not be obtainable during an exacerbation.
- Pulse oximetry may be useful for assessing the initial severity; a repeated measure of pulse oximetry of <92–94 percent after 1 hour is predictive of the need for hospitalization.
- Signs and symptoms scores may be helpful. Children who have signs and symptoms after 1–2 hours of initial treatment and who continue to meet the criteria for a moderate or severe exacerbation have a >84 percent chance of requiring hospitalization.
  — For adults:
- Repeated lung function measures (FEV_1 or PEF) at 1 hour and beyond are the strongest single predictor of hospitalization. Such measures may not be helpful, or easily obtained, during severe exacerbations.
- Pulse oximetry is indicated for patients who are in severe distress, have FEV_1 or PEF <40 percent predicted, or are unable to perform lung function measures. Only repeat assessments after initial treatment, not a single assessment upon admission, are useful for predicting the need for hospitalization.
- Signs and symptoms scores at 1 hour after initial treatments improve the ability to predict need for hospitalization. The presence of drowsiness is a useful predictor of impending respiratory failure and is reason to consider immediate transfer to a facility equipped to offer ventilatory support.

- **Consider adjunctive treatments, such as intravenous magnesium sulfate or heliox,** in severe exacerbations, if patients are unresponsive to the initial treatments listed above (e.g., FEV_1 or PEF <40 percent predicted or personal best after initial treatments).

- **Provide the following to prevent relapse of the exacerbation** and recurrence of another exacerbation:
  - Referral to followup asthma care within 1–4 weeks. In addition, encourage the patient to contact (e.g., by telephone) his/her asthma care provider during the first 3–5 days after discharge. A followup visit is essential to review the patient's written asthma action plan, adherence, and environmental control and to consider a step up in therapy. If appropriate, consider referral to an asthma self-management education program.
  - An ED asthma discharge plan. See figure 23a, b "Emergency Department—Asthma Discharge Plan."
  - Review of inhaler technique whenever possible.
  - Consideration of initiating ICS.

- **Treatments that are not recommended in the emergency care or hospital setting include:** methylxanthines, antobiotics (except as needed for comorbid conditions), aggressive hydration, chest physical therapy, mucolytics, or sedation. Inhaled ipratropium bromide is a helpful adjunctive therapy in the emergency care setting, but does not provide additional benefit after a patient is hospitalized for a severe exacerbation.

FIGURE 23a. EMERGENCY DEPARTMENT—ASTHMA DISCHARGE PLAN

EMERGENCY DEPARTMENT—ASTHMA DISCHARGE PLAN

Name: _____ was seen by Dr. _____ on ___/___/___

- Take your prescribed medications as directed—do not delay!
- _____-term treatment plan.
- Even when you feel well, you may need daily medicine to keep your asthma in good control and prevent attacks.
- Visit your doctor or other health care provider as soon as you can to discuss how to control your asthma and to develop *your own* action plan.

Your followup appointment with _____ is on: ___/___/___. Tel: _____

YOUR MEDICINE FOR THIS ASTHMA ATTACK IS:

Medication	Amount	Doses per day, for # days
Prednisone/prednisolone (oral corticosteroid)		____ a day for ____ days. Take the entire prescription, even when you start to feel better.
Inhaled albuterol		____ puffs every 4 to 6 hours if you have symptoms, for ____ days

YOUR DAILY MEDICINE FOR LONG-TERM CONTROL AND PREVENTING ATTACKS IS:

Medication	Amount	Doses per day
Inhaled corticosteroids		

YOUR QUICK-RELIEF MEDICINE WHEN YOU HAVE SYMPTOMS IS:

Medication	Amount	Number of doses/day
Inhaled albuterol		

ASK YOURSELF 2 TO 3 TIMES PER DAY, EVERY DAY, FOR AT LEAST 1 WEEK:

"How good is my asthma compared to when I left the hospital?"

If you feel much better:	If you feel better, but still need your quick-relief inhaler often:	If you feel about the same:	If you feel worse:
• Take your daily long-term control medicine.	• Take your daily long-term control medicine. • See your doctor as soon as possible.	• Use your quick-relief inhaler. • Take your daily long-term control medicine. • See your doctor as soon as possible—don't delay.	• Use your quick-relief inhaler. • Take your daily long-term control medicine. • Immediately go to the emergency department or call 9-1-1.

YOUR ASTHMA IS UNDER CONTROL WHEN YOU:

① Can be active daily and sleep through the night.	② Need fewer than 4 doses of quick-relief medicine in a week.	③ Are free of shortness of breath, wheeze, and cough.	④ Achieve an acceptable "peak flow" (discuss with your health care provider).

Reprinted by permission from Carlos Camargo, M.D., Principal Investigator of Agency for Health Care Research and Quality. Grant No. R13H31094.

Source: Camargo CA Jr, Emond SD, Boulet L, Gibson PG, Kolbe J, Wagner CW, Brenner BE. Emergency Department Asthma Discharge Plan. Developed at "Asthma Education in the Adult Emergency Department: A Multidisciplinary Consensus Conference," New York Academy of Medicine, New York, NY; 2001 April 1–5. Boston, MA: Massachusetts General Hospital, 2001. 2 pp.

FIGURE 23b. EMERGENCY DEPARTMENT—ASTHMA DISCHARGE PLAN: HOW TO USE YOUR METERED-DOSE INHALER

Using an inhaler seems simple, but most patients do not use it the right way. When you use your inhaler the wrong way, less medicine gets to your lungs.

For the next few days, read these steps aloud as you do them or ask someone to read them to you. Ask your doctor, nurse, other health care provider, or pharmacist to check how well you are using your inhaler.

Use your inhaler in one of the three ways pictured below (A or B are best, but C can be used if you have trouble with A and B). (Your doctor may give you other types of inhalers.)

Steps for Using Your Inhaler

Getting ready
1. Take off the cap and shake the inhaler.
2. Breathe out all the way.
3. Hold your inhaler the way your doctor said (A, B, or C below).

Breathe in slowly
4. As you start breathing in slowly through your mouth, press down on the inhaler one time. (If you use a holding chamber, first press down on the inhaler. Within 5 seconds, begin to breathe in slowly.)
5. Keep breathing in slowly, as deeply as you can.

Hold your breath
6. Hold your breath as you count to 10 slowly, if you can.
7. For inhaled quick-relief medicine (short-acting beta$_2$ agonists), wait about 15–30 seconds between puffs. There is no need to wait between puffs for other medicines.

A. Hold inhaler 1 to 2 inches in front of your mouth (about the width of two fingers).

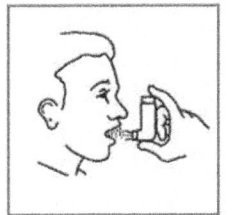

B. Use a spacer/holding chamber. These come in many shapes and can be useful to any patient.

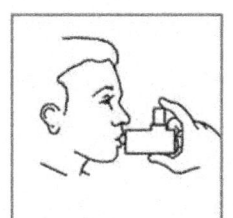

C. Put the inhaler in your mouth. Do not use for steroids.

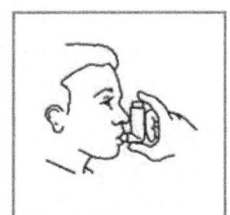

Clean your inhaler as needed, and know when to replace your inhaler. For instructions, read the package insert or talk to your doctor, other health care provider, or pharmacist.

For More Information

The National Heart, Lung, and Blood Institute (NHLBI) Health Information Center (HIC) is a service of the NHLBI of the National Institutes of Health. The NHLBI HIC provides information to health professionals, patients, and the public about the HIC treatment, diagnosis, and prevention of heart, lung, and blood diseases and sleep disorders. For more information, contact:

NHLBI Health Information Center
P.O. Box 30105
Bethesda, MD 20824-0105
Phone: 301-592-8573
TTY: 240-629-3255
Fax: 301-592-8563
Web site: http://www.nhlbi.nih.gov

DISCRIMINATION PROHIBITED: Under provisions of applicable public laws enacted by Congress since 1964, no person in the United States shall, on the grounds of race, color, national origin, handicap, or age, be excluded from participation in, be denied the benefits of, or be subjected to discrimination under any program or activity (or, on the basis of sex, with respect to any education program and activity) receiving Federal financial assistance. In addition, Executive Order 11141 prohibits discrimination on the basis of age by contractors and subcontractors in the performance of Federal contracts, and Executive Order 11246 States that no federally funded contractor may discriminate against any employee or applicant for employment because of race, color, religion, sex, or national origin. Therefore, the National Heart, Lung, and Blood Institute must be operated in compliance with these laws and Executive Orders.

Made in the USA
Coppell, TX
03 June 2020